D0929969

ELECTROCARDIOGRAMS
A SYSTEMATIC METHOD OF READING THEM

BY

MICHAEL L. ARMSTRONG, M.B., B.S.

WITH A FOREWORD BY

A. L. WINGFIELD, M.D., F.R.C.P.

Senior Physician, Seamen's Hospital, Greenwich, and Willesden General Hospital;
Honorary Cardiologist, St. Andrew's Hospital, Dollis Hill, London

SECOND EDITION

BALTIMORE: THE WILLIAMS AND WILKINS COMPANY
1968

© JOHN WRIGHT & SONS LTD., 1968

Library
I.U.P.
Indiana, Pa.
616.12 Au58e 2
c. 1

Distribution by Sole Agents:
United States of America: The Williams & Wilkins Company, Baltimore
Canada: The Macmillan Company of Canada Ltd., Toronto

First Edition, February, 1965

SBN 7236 0214 X

PRINTED IN GREAT BRITAIN BY JOHN WRIGHT & SONS LTD.
AT THE STONEBRIDGE PRESS, BRISTOL

PREFACE TO THE SECOND EDITION

FOR this edition I have rewritten almost the entire text although the original format remains unchanged. Most of the figures have been enlarged and clarified, and many have been replaced.

It has been my good fortune thus far to have worked with extremely knowledgeable colleagues, but, even more important, I have found these senior colleagues always helpful and eager to teach, encourage, and advise. I am therefore very pleased for this opportunity to thank Associate Professor John B. Hickie, M.B., B.S., M.R.C.P., F.R.A.C.P., F.A.C.C., for the pleasure of working with him over the past three years or so and for his very constructive help and advice with the present text.

Sydney   M. L. A.
1968

PREFACE TO THE FIRST EDITION

ELECTROCARDIOGRAPHY is not a new science, but unlike many other clinical investigations it is not open to experimental error, neither is it too dependent upon the technician who carries it out. It is a simple procedure and, like Mathematics, is an exact science dependent upon a knowledge of basic theorems for its interpretation.

I have not attempted here to discourse upon the underlying physiological and electrical theories of electrocardiography, but what I have attempted is to put down in as orderly a way as possible the facts which must be known and understood before any information can be gained from an electrocardiographic tracing.

In the second part of this small book I have tried to show that once these principles are known one should be able to look systematically at each component of the electrocardiogram and by a logical step-by-step procedure come to an exact diagnosis in a very short time.

There is nothing new or novel about this system, but unlike many speculative processes, it always pays dividends and is simple to use.

It is not very often that one has the chance to express one's gratitude publicly, so that I am very grateful for this opportunity to thank my adviser, teacher, and, in the true sense of the word, my friend, Dr. Alec Wingfield, M.D., F.R.C.P., for his considerable help and interest during the period in which it has been my good fortune to know him. More recently, I thank him for his suggestions and criticisms concerning this book and for writing the foreword.

I am also very indebted to Dr. Ewart Jepson, M.D., M.R.C.P., for his ready willingness to give advice, help, and support on so many occasions, and especially for the pleasure of working with him.

My gratitude also goes to Dr. Douglas Woolf, D.Phys.Med., and Dr. Freida Young, D.C.P., F.C.Path., whose help and friendship have been much appreciated.

Finally, I am indebted to Dr. David Weitzman, M.D., M.R.C.P., for the loan of some of the tracings reproduced herein, and I thank Mrs. W. Mitchell for mounting and collecting most of the other tracings, and Mrs. H. Hobbs and Mrs. F. L. Linsell for the typing.

M. L. A.

CONTENTS

FOREWORD

INTERPRETATION of electrocardiograms worries the newly qualified house-physician more than most aspects of the strange new world into which the transition from student to doctor plunges the holder of a first appointment. As a student, these tracings present an academic challenge, but in hospital practice a correct reading may make the difference between life and death, and frequently determines the correct line of treatment.

Dr. Armstrong has set himself the task of providing a logical sequence of observations which should lead with certainty towards correct diagnosis. What is novel in this book is the lucid approach to the subject and the inevitability of the conclusions to which this leads. He has described and illustrated the method which he himself used a few years ago and which, since then, he has passed on with great success to many others. This is neither a synopsis nor a complete textbook, but an exposition of a simple method, yet, in spite of this restriction, the reader will find in this volume almost everything of basic importance in the practical application of the electrocardiograph.

The illustrations are good and clear, and the text is free from ambiguity.

The author of this small book has proved what many already know, that those who have recently mastered a subject are best qualified to teach it to others. Many could have written this book, but very few could have done it better.

ALEC WINGFIELD

To
DIANE

—ELECTROCARDIOGRAMS—
A SYSTEMATIC METHOD OF READING THEM

CHAPTER I

INTRODUCTION

THE object of this book is not only to describe the electrocardiographic changes in various disease processes but to set out a method whereby anyone starting with a minimum of basic knowledge may be able to pick up an electrocardiographic tracing and by a logical step-by-step process arrive at the diagnosis or diagnoses.

The electrocardiograph is, in simple terms, a machine which measures the changes in electrical current, i.e., the electrical potential, between two points in the heart and records them on a previously sensitized paper. Preceding each cardiac contraction, excitation waves of electrical activity spread from the sino-atrial node through right and left atria to the atrioventricular node. After a short delay in electrical transmission while the ventricles fill with blood, the excitation wave passes along right and left branches of the bundle of His to the Purkinje system and the ventricles. The electrocardiograph utilizes the fact that when any muscle is stimulated, and in electrocardiography we are concerned with cardiac muscle, there is a change in electrical potential along the muscle-fibre. This change can be picked up by a galvanometer and the electrocardiograph is, in fact, basically a recording galvanometer.

It should be noted that the electrocardiogram must be interpreted in relationship to the clinical features of the patient and is no more than an aid to diagnosis, although considerable information can be derived from it.

Unipolar Leads.—The patient is connected to the machine by means of metal electrodes which are strapped on to the right and left arms and left leg. Wires from the machine are connected to each electrode. An electrode is also placed on the right leg, but this is not used for recording purposes and serves only to earth the patient. The negative side of the electrocardiograph is connected to a zero terminal and this zero terminal results from connecting leads from the three limbs to a central terminal. The central terminal is in turn connected to the gal-vanometer and the zero potential results because the potentials at the three points cancel one another out. These unipolar leads record the potential changes in a single electrode and are named as follows:—

Lead VR, which is the unipolar lead on the right arm and records the changes in potential occurring in that part of the heart facing the right shoulder, i.e., it is the electrical potential transmitted from this part of the heart to the right arm electrode.

1

Lead VL, which is the unipolar lead on the left arm and records the changes in potential in that part of the heart facing the left shoulder transmitted to the left-arm electrode.

Lead VF, which is the unipolar lead on the left leg and records the changes in potential in that part of the heart facing the left hip transmitted to the left-leg electrode.

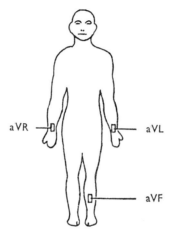

Fig. 1.—Standard augmented unipolar limb leads.

Unfortunately, these unipolar limb leads often have too low a voltage to be satisfactorily recorded; as a result, Goldberger devised a method whereby the deflexions can be increased in size, and these leads are therefore called *augmented unipolar limb leads* and are designated aVR, aVL, and aVF (*Fig.* 1). They are augmented by disconnecting the limb having the exploring electrode from the central zero terminal. This increases the voltage by 50 per cent.

When aVR, aVL, and aVF are all connected together, their combined potential is also zero, so that this combination can complete the electrical circuit but does not contribute to the record and can function as what is called an *indifferent electrode*.

Bipolar Leads.—As with any galvanometer, electrodes must be placed so as to enable difference in electrical potential to be picked up. The *standard limb leads* are bipolar. That is, the positive side of the electrocardiograph is connected to an electrode on one limb and the negative side of the machine is connected to an electrode on another limb, i.e., there are two poles, hence the term 'bipolar'. The bipolar leads are designated:—

Lead I, when the electrocardiograph is attached to the right and left arms and represents the difference in potential between these two points.

Lead II, when the electrocardiograph is attached to the right arm and left leg and represents the difference in potential between these two points.

Lead III, when the electrocardiograph is attached to the left leg and left arm and represents the difference in potential between these two points.

These three leads constitute the *standard* or *limb leads*.

2

Sometimes an extra lead, Lead IIIR, is taken with the selecting dial on the electrocardiograph pointing to Lead III but with the patient's chest held in full inspiration, so that the diaphragm is at its lowest point and the heart is brought closer to the chest wall and made more nearly vertical in position. Lead IIIR may exaggerate any changes in Lead III.

In actual fact, Leads III and aVF give a fair representation of electrical activity in the posterior part of the heart and are called *posterior limb leads*. However, small changes in Leads III and aVF are not always significant and can be very misleading.

Leads I and aVL are termed *anterior limb leads* and represent changes in electrical activity in the anterolateral aspect of the heart, especially in the left ventricle. The changes in Leads I and aVL often show corresponding changes in the chest leads V1–V6.

The Precordial or Superficial Chest Leads.—When these are taken, two electrodes are used. One electrode is placed in varying positions on the chest over the region of the heart and is called the 'exploring electrode'. The other electrode is the 'indifferent' electrode mentioned previously.

These electrodes transmit changes in electrical potential from the heart in the region of the exploring electrode.

There will obviously be some variations in the amplitude of deflexion on the electrocardiogram, depending on the distance of the exploring electrode from the heart and on the thickness of the chest wall. In thick-chested individuals, only a small amplitude of deflexion may occur, whereas, in thin-chested individuals, the amplitude of deflexion may be much greater.

The precordial leads are prefixed by the letter 'V' and their positions are shown on *Fig. 2*.

Lead V1 is taken with the electrode over the fourth intercostal space just to the right of the sternum.

Lead V2 is taken with the electrode over the fourth intercostal space just to the left of the sternum.

Lead V3 is taken with the electrode exactly midway between Leads V2 and V4.

Lead V4 is taken with the electrode in the midclavicular line over the fifth left intercostal space.

Lead V5 is taken with the electrode on the same level as V4, but in the anterior axillary line.

Lead V6 is taken with the electrode on the same level as V4 and V5, but in the midaxillary line.

Lead V7 is taken with the electrode on the same level as V4, V5, and V6, but in the posterior axillary line.

The Electrocardiographic Paper.—This is usually nowadays a long roll of paper with a coated carbon surface, and is composed of a number of 1- and 5-mm. squares (*Fig. 3*).

Vertically, these represent the amount of *electrical potential* involved in each electrocardiographic complex, and if the machine is correctly standardized, an impulse of 1 millivolt causes a deflexion of 10 mm.

3

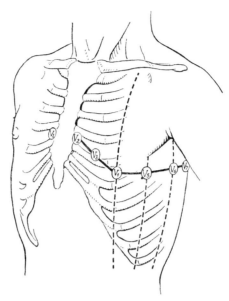

Fig. 2.—Positions of the exploring electrode on the chest wall.

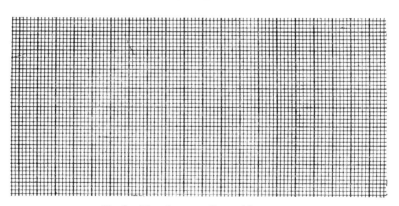

Fig. 3.—The electrocardiographic paper.

Horizontally, each millimetre represents a unit of *time*—0·04 sec.

It will be seen from *Fig.* 3 that the larger squares contain five of the single 1-mm. squares, thus each large square represents 5 mm. in vertical height and 5 multiplied by 0·04 sec. of time horizontally, i.e., 0·2 sec.

On most machines, the roll of paper moves at a constant rate of 25 mm. per sec., but on some machines the rate can be varied.

The Electrocardiographic Complex.—This is seen to be composed of a number of different waves together with the intervals between these waves (*Fig.* 4).

The P wave is the first wave and represents conduction through both right and left atria. The impulse is initiated in the sino-atrial node which is situated in the

4

right atrium and acts as the chief pacemaker of the heart. From here, the depolarization process travels through atrial musculature to the atrioventricular node.

The P *wave* is normally upright in most leads, but can be upright, diphasic, or inverted in Lead III, depending on the vector of travel during the process of auricular depolarization. It may be inverted in Leads aVr, aVL, and occasionally in Lead V1. The greatest amplitude is usually seen in Lead II. It is not usually higher than 2·5 mm. and its duration is not usually longer than 0·1 sec.

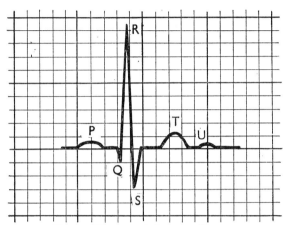

Fig. 4.—The normal electrocardiogram.

Sometimes the P waves are rather flat and ill defined, especially in an electrocardiogram of low voltage or when the cardiac rate increases sufficiently for the T–P interval to shorten until T and P waves become superimposed.

The QRS *complex* follows the P wave and the P–R interval, and represents ventricular depolarization. It is composed of a Q wave, an R wave, and an S wave, and the total duration should be measured in the limb lead in which it is longest.

The beginning of the QRS complex records activation of the interventricular septum, the left side being more markedly and more rapidly activated than the right. Next to be activated are the inner layers of both ventricles. The wave then spreads towards the outer layers of the ventricles.

When depolarization of the entire myocardium has occurred, there is a phase of recovery which begins with the S–T segment and is followed by the T wave which represents the major part of the recovery process.

The QRS complex is always inverted in Lead aVR which usually has a small or absent R wave. The normal duration of the QRS complex in adults is from 0·06 to 0·10 sec. and varies with cardiac rate and age, being shorter in children.

The Q *wave* may be absent. When present, it is defined as the first downward deflexion in the QRS complex if it is not preceded by an R or an S wave. (*Fig.* 4.) If there is only one negative deflexion, it is termed a QS wave.

Q waves occur normally in left ventricular surface leads such as Leads I, V4, V5, and V6. They are usually narrow with no notching or slurring, and are the result of septal activation.

The duration of the Q waves is usually less than 0·04 sec. and never lasts longer than 25 per cent of the total QRS complex duration. The depth of the Q wave is usually less than 2 mm. in Leads I and II and is rarely more than 1 mm. in depth in any of the other leads. A deeper Q wave may occur in Lead III in normal individuals, but it may also represent regressive changes of a postero-inferior myocardial infarct. However, in this situation, supporting evidence may be seen in Leads aVF and sometimes Leads V5 and V6.

Deep Q waves may occasionally occur in normal individuals in Lead V1, and more rarely in Lead V2.

The R *wave* is the first wave of the QRS complex deflected upwards, and its duration is usually less than 0·07 sec. Its amplitude varies considerably in normal people.

The S *wave* is the first downward deflexion following an R wave and is rarely deeper than 6 mm. S waves may sometimes be absent in all the standard limb leads.

The S–T *segment and the* T *wave* represent the process of recovery after ventricular contraction and may be followed by a small U wave. The S–T segment is measured from the end of the QRS complex to the beginning of the T wave. Its duration varies inversely with cardiac rate and usually ranges from nil to 0·15 sec.

The T *wave* usually starts on the iso-electric line and may have various shapes, ranging from tall and peaked through to flat, biphasic, and even inverted shapes. The T waves vary considerably in size, but are usually more than 2 mm. high and upright in all leads except Lead aVR. The T wave may be inverted in Lead III and in chest leads V1 and V2 in normal individuals. However, an inverted T wave in Leads I or II is usually abnormal.

The U *wave* represents the period of greatest excitability of the ventricle. It is most marked in Lead V3. It is frequently difficult to see and is usually upright in the limb and precordial leads and in the same direction as the T wave in most leads.

The P–R *interval* represents the time taken for electrical conduction from the sino-atrial node to ventricular muscle and is usually measured from the beginning of the P wave to the beginning of the QRS complex. Its duration varies normally from 0·10 to 0·20 sec.

The Q–T *interval* represents the total time taken for depolarization and re-polarization of ventricular muscle. It varies with age, sex, and cardiac rate and is measured in seconds. The maximum duration is 0·4 sec. for a cardiac rate of about 70 per min. For purposes of comparison, the Q–T interval must be corrected for variations in heart-rate and this is done by means of a formula (*see* p. 54).

It is helpful to note that in Lead V1 the R wave is usually small and the S wave deep, and as we pass across the chest, the R wave gradually increases in size and the S wave becomes smaller (*Fig. 5*).

Midway across the chest at about Lead V3, which corresponds with the site of the interventricular septum, the R and S waves are almost equal. By the time we have reached the lateral chest leads, the R wave has become quite tall, and the S wave has become almost non-existent.

The R wave in Lead V6 and the S wave in Lead V1 represent *left* ventricular activity and vice versa, i.e., the R wave in Lead V1 and the S wave in Lead V6 represent *right* ventricular activity.

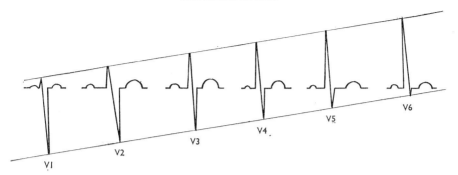

Fig. 5.—Diagram showing inverse relationship between R and S waves across the chest wall.

Clockwise and Anti-clockwise Rotation of the Heart.—If we view the heart from below, we see that chest lead V3 or V4 is approximately overlying the inter-ventricular septum, so that in either Lead V3 or Lead V4 the R wave will be of equal amplitude to the S wave (*Fig.* 6).

If there is clockwise rotation of the heart about its vertical axis, then the R and S waves will not become equal until we reach either Lead V5 or V6 (*Fig.* 7).

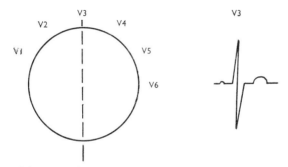

Fig. 6.—Diagram of the normal heart viewed from below with equal R and S waves in Lead V3.

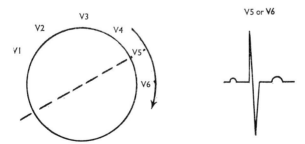

Fig. 7.—Diagram of clockwise rotation of heart with equal R and S waves in Lead V5.

On the other hand, if there is anti-clockwise rotation of the heart about its vertical axis, the R and S waves will become equal in amplitude in Leads V1 or V2 (*Fig.* 8).

7

Having thus some idea of what we are going to see when we have taken our tracing, we have only to connect up our patient to the machine and switch on. However, before taking the actual electrocardiogram, it is important to ensure correct standardization, so that different tracings may be compared on a similar

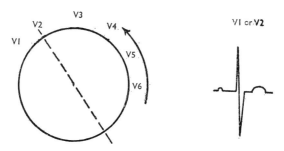

Fig. 8.—Diagram of anti-clockwise rotation of heart with equal R and S waves in Lead V1.

basis. This is usually carried out by pressure on a small knob on the machine which produces a standard deflexion equivalent to 1 millivolt. Each standardization deflexion should be mounted with the tracing for future reference and must be taken into account when interpreting the electrocardiogram. Many modern machines incorporate a control for halving the deflexion when very large complexes are present, as for example in gross left ventricular hypertrophy.

CHAPTER II

THE SYSTEMATIC APPROACH

THE few basic facts contained in the previous chapter must, of necessity, be fully understood before the prime purpose of this book is considered.

Taking for granted, then, that you are *au fait* with these premises, it remains only to consider the method of approach which should be used in the interpretation of all electrocardiograms.

There are many reference books both large and small about the subject of electrocardiography. However, I feel that if you have such a book, which usually describes each condition very well, you will, at the end, only be able to interpret your electrocardiogram if you happen to spot the abnormality on sight.

This seems to me to be a difficult and even hazardous procedure. *The object of this text is to teach a simple method whereby you may pick up any electrocardiogram and in a stage-by-stage process come to a complete diagnosis, be there one or many abnormalities.*

Each stage follows logically upon the one preceding it and EACH STAGE DEMANDS A DIAGNOSIS BEFORE PROCEEDING TO THE NEXT.

I will list the stages below.

Learn the order in which they come.

Stage I. The Rate.—
    If normal, proceed to Stage II.
    If rapid, why?
    If slow, why?

Stage II. The Rhythm.—
    If regular, proceed to Stage III.
    If irregular, why?

Stage III. Axis Deviation.—
    If left axis deviation is present, why?
    If right axis deviation is present, why?
    If neither is present, proceed to Stage IV.

Stage IV. The P Wave.—
    If normal, proceed to Stage V.
    If abnormal, why?

Stage V. The P–R Interval.—
    If normal, proceed to Stage VI.
    If abnormal, why?

Stage VI. The Q Wave.—
    If normal, proceed to Stage VII.
    If abnormal, why?

Stage VII. The QRS Complex.—
    If normal, proceed to Stage VIII.
    If abnormal, why?

Stage VIII. The Q–T Interval.—
    If normal, proceed to Stage IX.
    If abnormal, why?

Stage IX. The S–T Segment.—
    If normal, proceed to Stage X.
    If abnormal, why?

Stage X. The T Wave.—
    If abnormal, why?

These are the abnormalities and the order in which they will be considered:—

Stage I. The Rate.—
    IF RAPID.—
        1. Sinus tachycardia.
        2. Paroxysmal tachycardia.
            a. Supraventricular.
                i. Atrial.
                ii. Nodal.
            b. Ventricular.
        3. Atrial fibrillation.
        4. Atrial flutter.
        5. Ventricular fibrillation.
    IF SLOW.—
        1. Sinus bradycardia.
        2. Heart-block.
            a. First degree or latent. (This does not actually cause bradycardia.)
            b. Second degree or partial.
                i. With regular dropped beats.
                ii. With irregular dropped beats.
                iii. Wenckebach phenomenon.
            c. Third degree or complete.
        3. Sino-atrial block.
        4. Nodal rhythm.
    IF NORMAL.—
            a. Consider nodal rhythm.
            b. Consider normal electrocardiogram.

Stage II. The Rhythm.—
    IF REGULAR, ignore.
    IF IRREGULAR.—
        1. Sinus arrhythmia.
        2. Ectopic beats.
            a. Supraventricular.
                i. Atrial.
                ii. Nodal.

      b. Ventricular.
3. Atrial fibrillation.
4. Atrial flutter with variable heart block.
5. Ventricular fibrillation.
6. Variable heart-block.
7. Atrial tachycardia with irregular block.

Stage III. Axis Deviation.—
    IF LEFT AXIS DEVIATION.—Consider:—
      1. Left ventricular hypertrophy and dilatation.
      2. Rotation of the heart to the left.
      3. Left bundle-branch block.
      4. Horizontal heart.
    IF RIGHT AXIS DEVIATION.—Consider:—
      1. Right ventricular hypertrophy or dilatation.
      2. Rotation of the heart to the right.
      3. Right bundle-branch block.
      4. Vertical heart.
      5. Infants—and to a lesser extent children.
    IF NEITHER, ignore.

Stage IV. The P Wave.—
    IF NORMAL, ignore.
    IF ABNORMAL.—
      1. Absent P waves.
        a. Idioventricular rhythm.
        b. Atrial fibrillation.
      2. P pulmonale.
      3. P mitrale.
      4. Inverted P waves.
        a. Dextrocardia.
        b. Nodal rhythm.
        c. Sometimes physiological.
        d. Incorrectly placed arm leads.
      5. Multiple P waves.
        a. Atrial fibrillation (these are not strictly P waves).
        b. Atrial flutter.
        c. Atrial tachycardia with block.
        d. Heart-block.

Stage V. The P–R Interval.—
    IF NORMAL, ignore.
    IF ABNORMAL.—
      1. Prolonged P–R interval.
        a. Digitalis overdosage.
        b. First-degree heart-block.
        c. High serum potassium.

2. Short P–R interval.
   a. Wolff-Parkinson-White syndrome.
   b. Nodal rhythm.
3. Varying P–R interval—Wenckebach phenomenon.
4. P–R dissociation in third-degree heart-block.

Stage VI. The Q Wave.—
IF NORMAL, ignore.
IF ABNORMAL.—
   a. Myocardial infarction.
   b. Cardiomyopathy.

Stage VII. The QRS Complex.—
IF NORMAL, ignore.
IF ABNORMAL.—
   1. Widening of the QRS complex.
      a. Intraventricular conduction delay.
      b. Bundle-branch block.
         i. Right or left.
         ii. Complete or partial.
      c. High serum potassium.
      d. Ventricular ectopic beats.
      e. Quinidine.
      f. Ventricular hypertrophy.
   2. Low-voltage QRS complex.
      a. Obesity.
      b. Myocardial infarction.
      c. Chest diseases.
      d. Hypothyroidism.
      e. Pericardial effusion.
      f. Chronic constrictive pericarditis.
   3. Changes in shape.
      a. Slurring in bundle-branch block.
      b. In acute cor pulmonale, transient S waves and Q waves, S–T segment and aVR abnormalities.
      c. Abnormal configuration in myocardial infarction.
      d. Ventricular tachycardia.
      e. Ventricular fibrillation.
      f. Ventricular flutter.
      g. Variations in axis deviation.

Stage VIII. The Q–T Interval.—
IF NORMAL, ignore.
IF ABNORMAL.—
   1. Prolonged Q–T intervals.
      a. Hypocalcaemia.
      b. Active rheumatic carditis.
      c. Cardiac enlargement.

       d. Hypokalaemia.
       e. Ischaemic heart disease.
    2. Short Q–T intervals.
       a. Digitalis.
       b. High serum calcium.

Stage IX. The S–T Segment.—
    IF NORMAL, ignore.
    IF ABNORMAL.—
       1. Elevated S–T segment.
         a. Recent myocardial infarction.
         b. Pericarditis.
         c. Physiological.
         d. Cardiac trauma.
         e. Hyperkalaemia.
         f. Physiological.
       2. Depressed S–T segment.
         a. Ischaemia.
         b. Digitalis therapy.
         c. Tachycardia.
         d. Hypokalaemia.
         e. Ventricular hypertrophy.
         f. Bundle-branch block.
         g. Ectopic beats.

Stage X. The T Wave.—
    IF NORMAL, ignore.
    IF ABNORMAL.—
       1. Tall, peaked T waves.
         a. High serum potassium.
         b. In Leads V2 and V3 after posterior myocardial infarction.
       2. Flattened T waves.
         a. Myocardial ischaemia.
         b. Hypothyroidism.
         c. Pericarditis.
       3. Inverted T waves.
         a. Myocardial ischaemia.
         b. Pericarditis.
         c. Low serum potassium.
         d. Ventricular hypertrophy.

Stage XI. The U Wave.—
    IF NORMAL, ignore.
    IF ABNORMAL.—
       1. Prominent U wave.
         a. Ventricular hypertrophy.
         b. Bradycardia.
         c. Hypokalaemia.

13

       d. Hyperthyroidism.
       e. Digitalis.
       f. Adrenaline overdosage.
       g. Hypercalcaemia.
    2. Inverted U wave.
       a. Hyperkalaemia.
       b. Ischaemic heart disease.

We will now discuss each stage in detail.

STAGE I.—THE RATE

This is measured simply by counting the number of large, i.e., 5-mm., squares between corresponding waves of adjacent complexes and by dividing this number into 300. This gives the approximate rate per minute.

To ascertain *ventricular* rate, I think it easiest to take either the peaks of the R waves or the troughs of the S waves, as these are usually the most prominent.

Atrial rate is assessed by considering the number of large squares between consecutive P waves.

This method makes use of the fact that each of the heavy lines on the electrocardiographic paper is 0·2 sec. apart and there are 300 of these divisions per minute. (*Figs.* 9–12.)

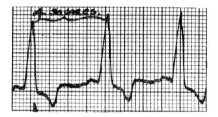

Fig. 9.—There are four large squares between corresponding waves in adjacent complexes, so that the rate $= \frac{300}{4} = 75$ beats per min.

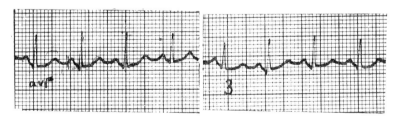

Fig. 10.—There are approximately two and a half large squares between corresponding components of adjacent complexes, so that the rate $= \frac{300}{2 \cdot 5} = 120$ beats per min.

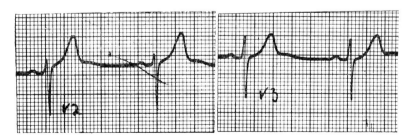

Fig. 11.—Rate $= \frac{300}{5 \cdot 6}$ approximately $= 54$ beats per min.

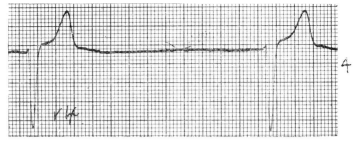

Fig. 12.—Rate = $\frac{300}{13}$ approximately = 23 beats per min.

If the rate is normal, e.g., between 60 and 90 beats per min., progress to Stage II, after a consideration of the possibility of nodal rhythm.

If the rate is rapid, consider the possible causes:—

      1. Sinus tachycardia.
      2. Paroxysmal tachycardia.
        a. Supraventricular.
          i. Atrial.
          ii. Nodal.
        b. Ventricular.
      3. Atrial fibrillation.
      4. Atrial flutter.
      5. Ventricular fibrillation.
      6. Ventricular flutter.

1. Sinus Tachycardia.—In this condition, the complexes are normal in every respect, but the rate is faster than 90 beats per min., and very rarely can reach up to 160 beats per min. Infants and children will almost invariably have sinus tachycardia. It may also be caused by: exercise; emotional stimuli of any type; congestive cardiac failure; blood or fluid loss; constrictive pericarditis; all the high output states, viz., fevers; anaemia; thyrotoxicosis; Paget's disease of bone;

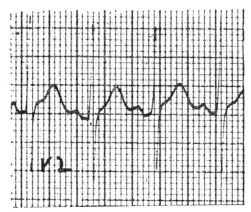

Fig. 13.—Rate = $\frac{300}{2}$ approximately = 150 beats per min. However, the P wave, P–R interval, and QRS complex are all normal. Sinus tachycardia.

16

advanced liver disease; anoxic cor pulmonale; beri-beri; and arteriovenous fistulae. (*Fig.* 13.) Carotid sinus pressure frequently produces gradual slowing of the cardiac rate, but the rhythm remains normal in sinus tachycardia.

2. Paroxysmal Tachycardia.—This is, in effect, a condition in which there is a series of ectopic beats which are usually rapid and which may be regular or irregular. The paroxysms usually begin and end abruptly.

Clinically, it is well recognized that paroxysmal tachycardia may present with the abrupt onset of palpitations, but it should also be remembered that severe tachycardia, whatever the type, may produce myocardial ischaemia and the patient may present with chest pain and shock, so mimicking the picture of myocardial infarction. If the rate is very rapid, it may produce syncope.

The site of origin of the ectopic beats determines the type of paroxysmal tachycardia. There are thus two main types:—

a. Supraventricular paroxysmal tachycardia may be either atrial or nodal and should be suspected if the rate is faster than 150 beats per min. and the rhythm is regular. The complexes are usually normal.

b. Ventricular paroxysmal tachycardia.

PAROXYSMAL ATRIAL TACHYCARDIA.—This is a series of rapid, regular, ectopic beats, arising from any focus in the atria other than the sino-atrial node.

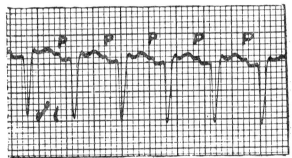

Fig. 14.—Rate $= \frac{300}{1 \cdot 6} = 187$ beats per min. However, P waves can be seen and the QRS complexes have a normal configuration. Atrial tachycardia.

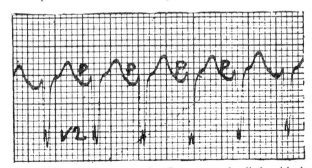

Fig. 15.—Rate $= \frac{300}{1 \cdot 6} = 187$ beats per min. P waves can be distinguished almost merged with the T waves. Note the notching of the S waves. This is due to a mechanical effect in the machine subsequent to the tachycardia. Atrial tachycardia.

17

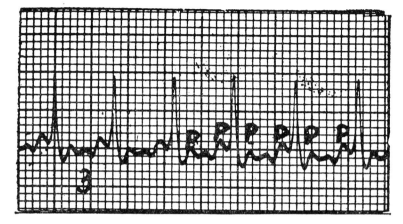

Fig. 16.—Rate $= \frac{300}{1\cdot6} = 187$ beats per min. The QRS complexes appear normal so that this is a supraventricular tachycardia. The configuration of the P waves appears to be normal. However, there are two P waves for every QRS complex. Atrial tachycardia with 2 : 1 atrioventricular block.

Atrial tachycardia is characterized on the electrocardiogram by:—

   i. A normal appearance of the QRS complex.

   ii. A rapid cardiac rate which is usually greater than 150 beats per min.

   iii. Difficulty in finding the P waves which may be merged with the rest of the complex.

   iv. Carotid sinus pressure causes a rise in vagal tone, which often abruptly terminates paroxysmal supraventricular tachycardia, as may other similar measures such as eyeball pressure, vomiting, gag reflex, etc.

The P waves, when they can be made out, are usually abnormal because they originate outside their usual focus of origin in the sino-atrial node. Their shape depends on the actual site of origin.

Clinically, it may sometimes be difficult to differentiate supraventricular tachycardia from atrial flutter with 2 : 1 atrioventricular block, and in these cases vagal stimulation may help by slowing down the rate in atrial flutter, whereas in supraventricular tachycardia carotid sinus pressure either has no effect or abolishes the tachycardia altogether.

Paroxysmal atrial tachycardia may be found in young people with no other cardiac abnormality. It is also said to be associated with tobacco, alcohol, and over-eating, and also occurs in rheumatic valve disease, especially mitral valve disease; ischaemic heart disease; atrial septal defect; and digitalis overdosage. (*Figs.* 14–16.)

PAROXYSMAL NODAL TACHYCARDIA.—This is less common than the atrial variety. The initiating focus is in the atrioventricular node.

If the rate is very fast, nodal tachycardia may be difficult to differentiate from the atrial type and a diagnosis of supraventricular tachycardia must suffice, because in both types the QRS complexes are almost normal.

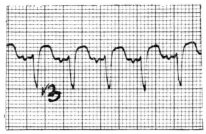

Fig. 17.—Rate more than 150 beats per min. Note the deformed P waves. Nodal tachycardia.

Less rapid bursts of paroxysmal nodal tachycardia are seen to have an inverted or in some other way deformed P wave which may occur either before, mixed with, or after the QRS complex. I would emphasize that the QRS complex in both forms of a supraventricular paroxysmal tachycardia is almost normal.

If there is retrograde conduction, the P waves are inverted in Leads II and III, or they may be entirely absent if there is no retrograde conduction. (*Fig.* 17.)

PAROXYSMAL VENTRICULAR TACHYCARDIA.—This is uncommon and is manifested on the electrocardiogram by bursts of bizarre QRS complexes in rapid succession.

This is easy to differentiate from the supraventricular forms of paroxysmal tachycardia because the QRS complexes look quite abnormal and bizarre. They are often wide and resemble the appearance in bundle-branch block (*see* p. 46). In some cases we may see P waves which are quite independent of the QRS complexes and which may have a much slower rate.

It may be difficult to differentiate paroxysmal ventricular tachycardia from atrial tachycardia with bundle-branch block.

Paroxysmal ventricular tachycardia may present clinically in similar ways to the supraventricular forms, but it suggests much more serious cardiac damage.

It is associated with: hypertensive cardiac disease; myocardial infarction; aortic valve disease; digitalis therapy; and diphtheritic carditis.

It may sometimes succeed a Stokes-Adams attack. In some cases, it may be innocent. Clinically, paroxysmal ventricular tachycardia may resemble supraventricular tachycardia apart from its failure to respond to carotid sinus pressure

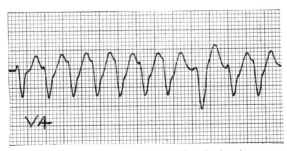

Fig. 18.—Rate approximately 250 beats per min. The rhythm is not completely regular and the complexes are bizarre in form. Paroxysmal ventricular tachycardia.

19

and cholinergic drugs. There may also be some variation in the fifth heart-sound. Not infrequently, it is followed by ventricular fibrillation and sudden death. Frequently, it precipitates congestive cardiac failure. (*Fig.* 18.)

3. Atrial Fibrillation.—This is a condition in which, as the name suggests, the atria are fibrillating, that is, they are beating irregularly and inefficiently and usually at a very rapid rate, often between 350 and 550 beats per min.

On the electrocardiogram we see that the ventricular rate, i.e., the frequency of the QRS complexes, is completely irregular and we will often see, in some

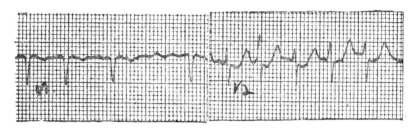

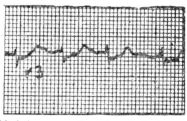

Fig. 19.—The rate is rapid, being approximately 100 beats per min., but is completely irregular. 'f' waves are best seen in Lead V1. Atrial fibrillation.

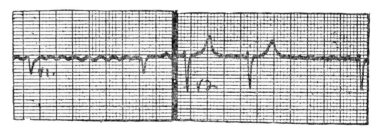

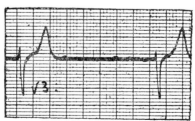

Fig. 20.—Atrial fibrillation. The ventricular rate is slow (it has been well controlled with digitalis) but is completely irregular. Classic 'f' waves may be seen in Lead V1.

20

leads at least, rapid and irregular atrial waves, called 'f' waves or fibrillation waves.

These are best seen in the precordial leads and may be large or small. They are, on occasion, difficult to define.

The atrial rate can be as high as 600 beats per min., and since the atrioventricular bundle is not able to conduct so rapidly and the ventricles are thus unable to respond, there must be some degree of atrioventricular dissociation or block.

It should be noted that with digitalis therapy, although the rate may be slowed, atrial fibrillation may still exist. In this circumstance the QRS complexes will still be completely irregular and 'f' waves may still be seen (*Fig.* 20).

Atrial fibrillation is best seen in: mitral stenosis; thryotoxicosis; ischaemic heart disease; hypertensive heart disease; constrictive pericarditis; congenital heart disease especially atrial septal defects; and sometimes in patients with no other obvious heart disease. (*Figs.* 19, 20.)

4. Atrial Flutter.—This is the result of a regular flow of impulses from some irritable focus in atrial muscle. However, unlike atrial fibrillation, the discharge of impulses is quite regular and may be up to 350 per min. These flutter or 'F' waves resemble, in profile, the teeth of a saw and hence give rise to the typical so-called 'saw-tooth' appearance. (*Fig.* 22.)

As in atrial fibrillation, the ventricles may be unable to respond to so rapid an atrial rate, so that there will often be some degree of atrioventricular block.

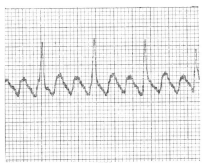

Fig. 21.—Atrial flutter. Ventricular rate is almost 100 beats per min. 2 : 1 regular atrioventricular block.

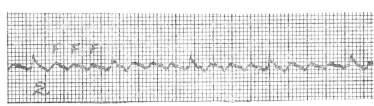

Fig. 22.—Atrial flutter with characteristic 'F' waves of saw-tooth appearance. The ventricular rate is approximately 75 beats per min. There are four 'F' waves to each ventricular complex, the atrial rate being about 300 per min. Atrial flutter with 4 : 1 atrioventricular block.

Usually, however, the ventricles respond to every other atrial beat, i.e., there will be two flutter waves to every ventricular complex with a resulting 2 : 1 block. Sometimes, 3 : 1 and even 4 : 1 block may occur and the degree of block can even vary in different leads and less commonly in the same lead, so that the rhythm may become irregular.

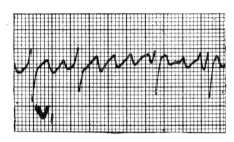

Fig. 23.—Atrial flutter with variable block, 4 : 1 and 2 : 1.

Clinically, atrial flutter may present, as may the other forms of tachycardia, with angina pectoris and may sometimes precipitate congestive cardiac failure. It can resemble any of the paroxysmal tachycardias in its abrupt onset, but it tends to last longer. Differentiation may be aided by carotid sinus pressure which may slow the ventricular rate and thus increase the atrioventricular block in atrial flutter but may not affect paroxysmal tachycardia.

It is important to note that atrial flutter is very uncommonly seen in Lead I, and is best seen in Leads II and III aVR, aVF, and V1. Atrial flutter is usually associated with organic heart disease and occurs especially in: rheumatic heart disease; ischaemic heart disease; hypertensive heart disease; cor pulmonale. (*Figs.* 21–23.)

5. Ventricular Fibrillation.—This occurs in advanced cardiac disease and may follow cardiac arrest, electric shock, or digitalis intoxication.

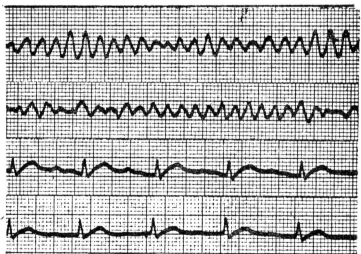

Fig. 24.—Ventricular fibrillation reverting to sinus rhythm with occasional ectopic beats after defibrillation.

22

It is due to the presence in the ventricles of irritable foci which discharge impulses irregularly throughout the ventricular muscle.

The electrocardiogram shows bursts of completely irregular, bizarre and atypical complexes.

Sudden death usually ensues, but spontaneous recovery can occur and electrical defibrillation may produce resumption of sinus rhythm. Ventricular fibrillation may follow: cardiac arrest; adrenaline therapy; digitalis; chloroform administration; asphyxia; and advanced cardiac disease of almost any origin. (*Fig.* 24.)

Table I.—Some Differentiating Points

	Rate	Rhythm	First Heart-Sound	Carotid sinus Pressure
Sinus tachycardia	100–150	Regular	++Constant	Gradual slowing
Supraventricular tachycardia	140–240 (180–190)	Regular	++Constant	No effect or stops abruptly
Atrial flutter	120–180 (160)	Regular	Constant but changes with treatment	Abrupt slowing to half, jerky return to original rate
Ventricular tachycardia	150–250	Irregular	Varying	No effect

The above cases must be considered if the cardiac rate is rapid. However, if the rate is slow, the conditions to be considered are:—

    1. Sinus bradycardia.
    2. Complete heart-block.
    3. Nodal rhythm.

1. Sinus Bradycardia.—Apart from the fact that the cardiac rate is slow, i.e., less than 60 beats per min., the electrocardiographic complexes are completely normal in every respect. It is due to the fact that impulses are being discharged from the sino-atrial node, which is the normal cardiac pacemaker, at a slower rate than normal. It is found in: normal people; athletes; digitalis administration; hypothyroidism; jaundice; convalescence from infective fevers; raised intracranial pressure; and drugs such as reserpine. (*Fig.* 25.)

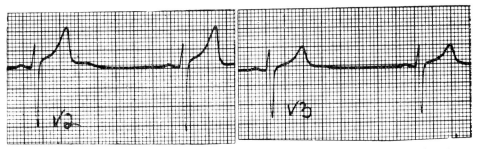

Fig. 25.—Rate is approximately 37 beats per min. The P waves, P–R intervals, and QRS complexes are all normal. Sinus bradycardia.

In hypothyroidism, as well as the presence of sinus bradycardia there is often an associated low electrical potential, i.e., the complexes are of small amplitude. (*See Figs.* 47, 64.)

2. Heart-block.—Several different conditions are frequently discussed incorrectly in a consideration of heart-block. More correctly, the term 'heart-block' implies only atrioventricular block, but some authors collectively discuss 'heart-block' under the following sub-headings:—

I. SINO-ATRIAL BLOCK.—Which suggests failure of the normal impulse to be discharged from the pacemaker or sino-atrial node. If there is complete sino-atrial block, there results bradycardia, because the sino-atrial node fails to discharge impulses altogether and another pacemaker takes over, often within the atrioventricular node, but sometimes within the ventricular muscle itself. The electrocardiographic appearances are of a slow atrioventricular nodal rhythm with delayed retrograde atrial stimulation from the new pacemaker.

On occasions, the block may be 'intermittent' with some impulses failing intermittently to be discharged from the sino-atrial node.

Sometimes, the delay in atrial excitation may be long enough to allow the atrial impulse to reactivate the atrioventricular conducting system, so that a second ventricular contraction occurs. This is called 'coupling' or 'bigeminus' (*see* p. 30).

II. ATRIOVENTRICULAR BLOCK.—In which there is dissociation between atrial and ventricular complexes. There are three grades of atrioventricular heart-block:—

a. LATENT OR FIRST-DEGREE HEART-BLOCK.—This is manifested on the electrocardiogram by a prolonged P–R interval.

The normal P–R interval ranges between 0·12 and 0·22 sec., i.e., from 3 to 5½ of the small (1-mm.) squares on the electrocardiographic paper.

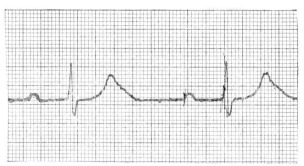

Fig. 26.—P–R interval 0·44 sec. The complexes are otherwise normal. First-degree or latent heart-block.

A P–R interval of longer than 0·22 sec. is taken as representing first-degree or latent heart-block. In extreme cases, the P–R interval may be above 0·32 sec. and may even coincide with the T wave of the previous complexes.

First-degree heart-block may be due to:—

i. Any form of active carditis, especially rheumatic.

24

Library
I.U.P.
Indiana, Pa.

ii. Pulmonary artery thrombosis.

iii. Fibrosis of the myocardium subsequent to ischaemia.

iv. Digitalis therapy.

v. Hypokalaemia.

vi. Carotid sinus pressure. (*Fig.* 26.)

b. PARTIAL OR SECOND-DEGREE HEART-BLOCK.—This implies that some atrial beats are not followed by the normal ventricular beat. That is, on the electrocardiogram each P wave may not always be followed by a QRS complex. However, it is important to note that where there *is* a QRS complex, it is preceded by a normal P wave and a normal and constant P–R interval.

Partial or second-degree heart-block may take one of three forms:—

i. Irregularly dropped beats but with a constant P–R interval, as discussed above.

ii. Regularly dropped beats resulting in a fixed atrioventricular relationship, e.g., 2 : 1, 3 : 1, or occasionally 4 : 1 heart-block (*Fig.* 27).

Here again, each QRS complex will be preceded by a constant P–R interval. This condition is found in: ischaemic heart disease; digitalis intoxication; less often in myocarditis, especially rheumatic and diphtheritic.

iii. The Wenckebach phenomenon, in which the P–R interval gradually lengthens before each ensuing QRS complex until gradually conduction fails and a beat is dropped. The next beat has a short P–R interval which once again gradually lengthens until again another beat is dropped and the cycle is repeated. This may be transient and recover spontaneously, but it can occasionally progress to complete heart-block. (*Fig.* 28.)

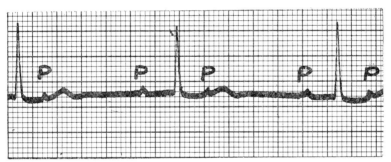

Fig. 27.—There are two P waves for each QRS complex, but each complex is preceded by a constant P–R interval. Partial or second-degree heart-block with regularly dropped beats.

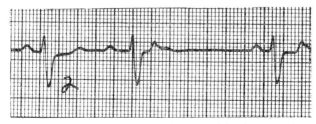

Fig. 28.—Gradual prolongation of the P–R interval with subsequent dropped beat. Wenckebach phenomenon.

25

3

c. COMPLETE OR THIRD-DEGREE HEART-BLOCK.—Here, the atria and the ventricles are beating quite independently of one another, that is, in the electrocardiogram the P waves bear no relationship to the QRS complexes at all and in each complex the P–R interval will be quite different. In some cases, the QRS complexes may be normal but are frequently a little deformed and widened.

The ventricular rate is usually very slow and is based on the inherent property of the ventricles to beat at their own, or idioventricular, rate, which is usually less than 40 beats per min.

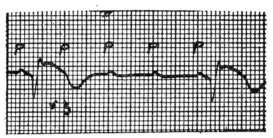

Fig. 29.—The ventricular rate is 37½ beats per min. For each QRS complex there are four P waves and each P–R interval is different. Complete 4 : 1 heart-block.

It is possible, although rare, for complete atrioventricular block to be present with quite a rapid ventricular rate.

Complete heart-block is most often found in: ischaemic heart disease; hypertensive heart disease; digitalis therapy; calcification in the bundle of His or its branches. This is associated with syphilitic aortitis and mitral or aortic sclerosis.

The main points, electrocardiographically speaking, in heart-block are that in *partial atrioventricular block there is a constant* P–R *interval* (except in the Wenckebach phenomenon) whereas *in complete heart-block there is no constant relationship between the* P *waves and the* P–R *intervals* in each complex and *each* P–R *interval of each complex will be different.* (*Figs.* 29, 30.)

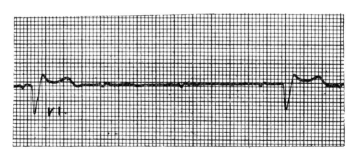

Fig. 30.—Complete 3 : 1 heart-block.

III. BUNDLE-BRANCH BLOCK.—Implies a disturbance through the conducting pathways of the bundle of His and will be dealt with later, under abnormalities of the QRS complex (*see* p. 46). It has no effect on cardiac rate.

3. Nodal Rhythm.—Sometimes, nodal rhythm can give rise to a bradycardia. Under normal conditions the sino-atrial node is the cardiac pacemaker, i.e., it is the site of origin of the electrical impulse which results in the cardiac cycle and hence the normal P–QRST complex of the electrocardiogram. Under some circumstances, the atrioventricular node may take over the functions of the sino-atrial node and so become the effective cardiac pacemaker, and since the

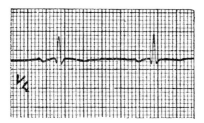

Fig. 31.—The rate is 60 beats per min. Note the deformed P waves. Nodal rhythm.

atrioventricular node initiates its impulses at a slower rate than the sino-atrial node, there will often be a resulting bradycardia.

This situation is termed 'nodal rhythm', and under these conditions the P wave may be inverted or in some other way deformed, because the excitation is retrograde, i.e., from the atrioventricular node towards the atria and sino-atrial node. The P wave may precede, coincide with, or follow the QRS complex, or may be absent altogether, and occasionally it may shift from moment to moment, because not uncommonly in nodal rhythm the ventricles receive their electrical impulse before the atria. Clinically, nodal rhythm can be recognized from its effect on the jugular venous pulse, because it is associated with sharp cannon waves. It is frequently a harmless rhythm change giving rise to no symptoms and requiring no therapy.

The commonest cause of nodal rhythm is digitalis therapy. However, it is also found in: active carditis, especially rheumatic and diphtheritic; thrombosis of the branch of the coronary artery supplying the sino-atrial node; normal individuals. (*Fig.* 31.)

Having considered the possible causes for the cardiac rate being either excessively fast or slow, we must next consider the second step in the interpretation of the electrocardiogram.

27

STAGE II.—THE RHYTHM

Look at every lead. If the rhythm is regular, pass on to Stage III; if not, consider the possible causes. They are:—

1. Sinus arrhythmia.
2. Ectopic beats.
    a. Supraventricular.
       i. Atrial.
      ii. Nodal.
    b. Ventricular.
3. Atrial fibrillation.
4. Atrial flutter with variable heart-block.
5. Ventricular fibrillation.
6. Variable heart-block.
7. Atrial tachycardia with irregular block.

1. Sinus Arrhythmia.—Not all normal hearts beat completely regularly, so that in some electrocardiograms we may see short episodes of slightly increased cardiac rate which gradually slow down. These changes may recur from time to time. However, the complexes are perfectly normal.

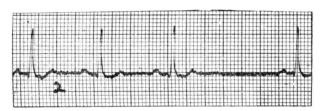

Fig. 32.—Sinus arrhythmia.

This is so-called 'sinus arrhythmia' and consists of an increase in cardiac rate during inspiration, often followed by slowing during expiration. It is due to alterations in vagal tone mediated by pressor receptors in the lungs and usually has no clinical significance. (*Fig.* 32.)

2. Ectopic Beats.—These are due to impulses being discharged from some ectopic focus which may be in the atria, the atrioventricular node, or in the ventricles. All are in fact so-called 'premature beats' in that they arrive earlier than they should in the cardiac cycle. A compensatory pause usually follows each ectopic beat.

There are three types of ectopic beats which correspond with the types of paroxysmal tachycardia. They are:—

a. ATRIAL ECTOPIC BEATS.—These arise from an irritable focus somewhere in the atria. The impulse then passes along the normal conductive pathways via the bundle of His.

28

In the electrocardiogram the P wave will be inverted or in some other way abnormal. It is followed by an almost normal QRS complex. (*Fig.* 33.)

Occasionally, atrial ectopic beats may precede atrial fibrillation, especially in mitral stenosis and thyrotoxicosis.

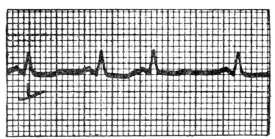

Fig. 33.—An atrial ectopic beat. Note the P waves and the compensatory pause.

b. NODAL ECTOPIC BEATS.—These arise in the atrioventricular node. Again, the QRS complex is normal or nearly so, and again, the P wave may be inverted. However, in nodal ectopic beats, as in nodal rhythm, the P wave may

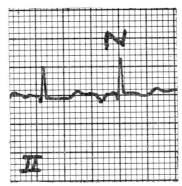

Fig. 34.—A nodal ectopic beat. Note the inverted P wave.

occur before, within, or after the QRS complex, so that in some cases no P wave may be discernible. (*Fig.* 34.)

c. VENTRICULAR ECTOPIC BEATS.—These are usually easy to diagnose on the electrocardiogram. There is no preceding P wave, since the beat arises from

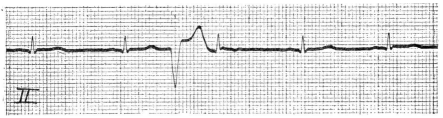

Fig. 35.—A typical ventricular ectopic beat which is bizarre and quite different from the other QRS complexes.

ventricular tissues. The QRS complex has a bizarre form which is quite different from other complexes in the same lead and is often widened and enlarged and thus resembles to some extent the pattern in bundle-branch block (*see* p. 46). As with supraventricular ectopic beats there is usually a compensatory pause following the ectopic beat.

One can often pinpoint the site of ventricular ectopic beats. If the complex resembles a *left* bundle-branch block, then the ectopic focus from which it arises is probably situated in the *right* ventricle and vice versa. (*Fig.* 35.)

BIGEMINUS OR COUPLING.—When each ventricular ectopic beat is closely related to a normal beat, the term 'bigeminus' or 'coupling' is used. This may be felt at the radial pulse and is seen especially in digitalis therapy. (*Fig.* 36.)

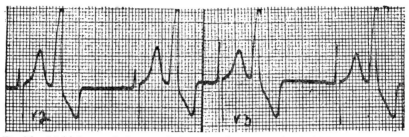

Fig. 36.—Multiple ventricular ectopic beats can be seen, each of which is quite bizarre in form. Note that each one is closely associated with or coupled to a normal ventricular complex. Bigeminus.

3. Atrial Fibrillation has already been discussed on p. 20.

4. Atrial Flutter with Variable Heart-block.—Atrial flutter with *fixed* atrioventricular block has been discussed previously (*see* p. 21).

However, occasionally the degree of atrioventricular block *may vary* even in the same lead and there will result a completely irregular tracing. (*See Fig.* 23, p. 22.)

5. Ventricular Fibrillation.

6. Variable Heart-block.
These conditions have already been discussed above.

Having considered the diagnosis in each of the first two stages of electrocardiographic interpretation, we now proceed to the third stage.

STAGE III.—AXIS DEVIATION

Every heart has an anatomical and an electrical axis. We are here primarily concerned with the *electrical axis*, which represents the direction of conduction of electrical impulses through the heart and is best represented by a vector force projected to the frontal plane. It usually lies between 0 and 90°, which is more or less the anatomical axis.

Left Axis Deviation.—In most normal hearts, the electrical axis is in the direction shown in *Fig.* 37.

If the heart rotates anatomically around its anteroposterior axis in an anti-clockwise direction as seen from the front (*Fig.* 38), then the *electrical axis* will also be seen to have rotated in the same direction. This may occur in obese individuals

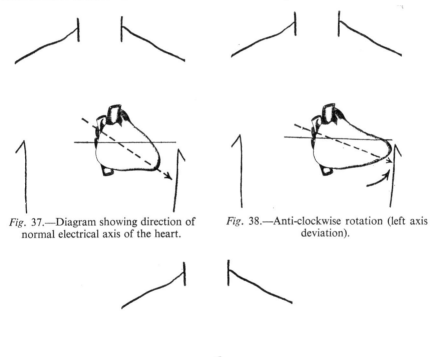

Fig. 37.—Diagram showing direction of normal electrical axis of the heart.

Fig. 38.—Anti-clockwise rotation (left axis deviation).

Fig. 39.—Anti-clockwise rotation (left axis deviation) due to left ventricular enlargement.

31

with an elevated left diaphragm or as a result of cardiac displacement to the left from scoliosis.

Similarly, if the left ventricle becomes enlarged with a resulting increase in electrical activity, then the electrical axis will again rotate in an anti-clockwise direction. (*Fig.* 39.)

Left axis deviation also occurs in 10 per cent of normal individuals.

It will be seen that in both conditions the *electrical axis* has rotated towards the left, and this is termed *left axis deviation*. It is also obvious from the diagrams that this electrical axis has moved towards a more horizontal plane. Hence the term *horizontal heart* which is often used as a synonym.

In other words, left axis deviation occurs in both left ventricular hypertrophy or enlargement *and* in anti-clockwise rotation of the heart about its anteroposterior diameter.

It should be noted that these two conditions may occur together or, of course, independently.

Left axis deviation may also be present in the uncommon form of atrial septal defect known as the 'ostium primum' type.

THE ELECTROCARDIOGRAM IN LEFT AXIS DEVIATION.—There are many ways of determining axis deviation. I think the simplest method is to look at limb leads I and III and in each of these two leads to determine the direction of greatest deflexion.

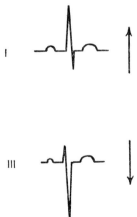

Fig. 40.—The electrocardiogram in left axis deviation.

Left axis deviation is said to be present when the direction of greatest deflexion in Lead I is upwards (i.e., when the R wave is the largest of the QRS complex); *and* the direction of greatest deflexion in Lead III is downwards (i.e., when the S wave is the largest of the QRS complex).

Put more simply: left axis deviation is present when the main direction of the QRS *complex points upwards in Lead I and downwards in Lead III, i.e., if Leads I and III diverge away from one another.* (*Fig.* 40.)

If left axis deviation does exist, we must look for left ventricular hypertrophy and for this we must examine the chest leads V1 to V6.

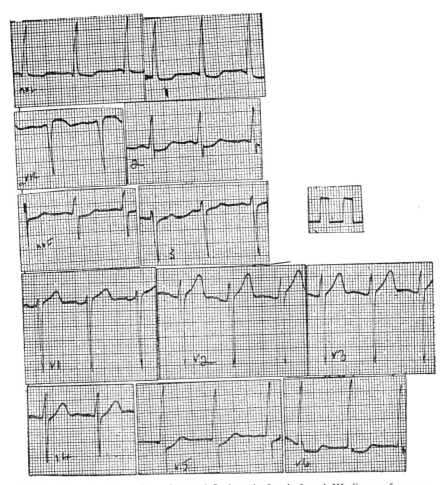

Fig. 41.—The directions of maximum deflexions in Leads I and III diverge from one another. Left axis deviation. We therefore look for left ventricular hypertrophy. The S wave in V1 is 24 mm. deep. The R wave in V6 is 24 mm. high. The sum of S in V1 and R in V6 is 48 mm., which is more than the required 35 mm. necessary to make a diagnosis of left ventricular hypertrophy. So this tracing shows left axis deviation and left ventricular hypertrophy.

LEFT VENTRICULAR HYPERTROPHY.—If the left ventricle hypertrophies, then there will be more electrical activity over it with corresponding elevation in potential difference, and the left ventricular component of the complex will become more prominent. Thus, the R waves in leads overlying the left ventricle (i.e., Leads V5 and V6) will become taller and, similarly, the S waves in Leads V1 and V2 will become deeper.

Left ventricular hypertrophy is therefore said to be present if the height of the R wave measured in millimetres in Lead V6 is added to the depth of the S wave measured in millimetres in Leads V1 or V2, and if the total is 45 mm. or more.

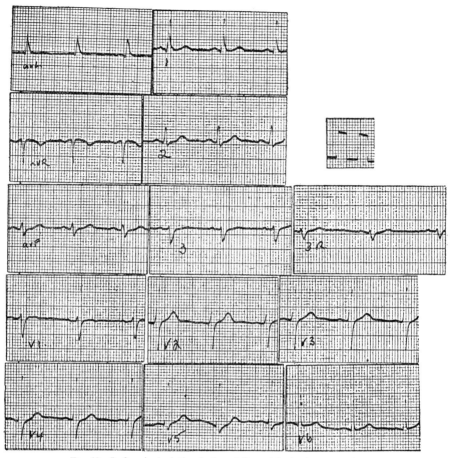

Fig. 42—Left axis deviation but no left ventricular hypertrophy.

It is also said to be present if S in V2 plus R in V5 equals 45 mm. or more; or if S in V1 plus R in V5 equals 38 mm. or more; or if S in V2 plus R in V6 equals 38 mm. or more. Left axis deviation is not always present in left ventricular hypertrophy.

In some cases of left ventricular hypertrophy, there may also be changes in the S–T segment or the T wave, the T wave being inverted and the S–T segment being depressed in chest leads V5 and V6. There may also be tall, upright T waves with an elevated S–T segment in Leads V1 and V2. (*Figs.* 41, 42.)

Occasionally, the normal semi-vertical position is maintained and this situation is called 'concordant left ventricular hypertrophy' and occurs characteristically in aortic stenosis.

Note that there may also be corresponding voltage changes in thick- or thin-chested individuals.

Right Axis Deviation.—If there is right ventricular enlargement, the electrical axis will change its direction towards the right (*Fig.* 43), and right axis deviation will exist. This will, of course, also occur if there is rotation of the heart around its anteroposterior diameter in a clockwise direction as in thin asthenic individuals (*Fig.* 44).

In both conditions, the *electrical axis* is seen to be approaching the vertical, hence the term *vertical heart*.

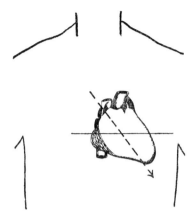

Fig. 43.—Right axis deviation due to right ventricular enlargement.

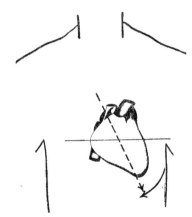

Fig. 44.—Right axis deviation in a thin asthenic individual.

Right axis deviation may also be present in acute cor pulmonale.

THE ELECTROCARDIOGRAM IN RIGHT AXIS DEVIATION.—Is best checked, as is *left* axis deviation, in limb leads I and III.

The direction of greatest deflexion of the QRS complex in Lead I is downwards, and in Lead III is upwards, i.e., these two leads converge towards one another, as in *Figs.* 45, 46.

If right axis deviation exists, we look for right ventricular hypertrophy (remembering that the cause may be only a long narrow chest).

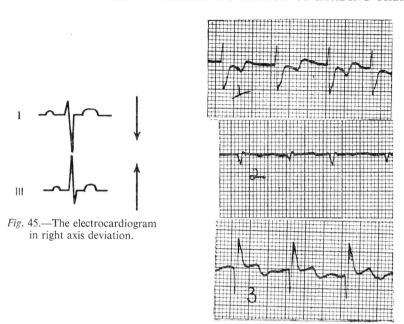

I

III

Fig. 45.—The electrocardiogram
in right axis deviation.

Fig. 46.—Right axis deviation in a case of massive pulmonary embolus.

RIGHT VENTRICULAR HYPERTROPHY.—To diagnose right ventricular hypertrophy we look at the limb leads, which show right axis deviation. In the chest leads V1 and V2 there will be a tall R wave, whilst in Leads V5 and V6 there will be a deep S wave.

Sometimes after a small initial septal R wave, there is a tall secondary R wave which replaces the usual S wave in Leads V1 and V2.

Secondary inversion of the T wave with slight depression of the R–T segment is common in Leads V1–V3.

Unlike left ventricular hypertrophy, in right ventricular hypertrophy there is no accepted numerical criterion above which we can say right ventricular hypertrophy exists.

Having considered the first three stages in the interpretation of our electro-cardiogram, we pass on to Stage IV.

36

STAGE IV.—THE P WAVE

Examine the P wave in every complex. If it is normal, pass on to Stage V; if abnormal, consider the possible reasons:—

1. Absent P waves.—
   a. Idioventricular rhythm.
   b. Atrial fibrillation.
2. P pulmonale.
3. P mitrale.
4. Inverted P waves.—
   a. Dextrocardia.
   b. Nodal rhythm.
   c. Incorrectly placed arm leads.
   d. Physiological.
5. Multiple P waves.—
   a. Atrial flutter.
   b. Atrial fibrillation. (These are not strictly P waves.)
   c. Atrial tachycardia with atrioventricular block.
   d. Heart-block.

The P wave is due to conduction and spread of the electrical impulse from the sino-atrial node to the atrioventricular node through right and left atria. It is not usually higher than 2·5 mm., but may be much smaller and does not usually last for longer than 0·1 sec. Sometimes it may be very small and difficult to define.

The P waves are usually upright in all the standard limb leads and are usually greatest in Lead II.

Occasionally, the P wave may be inverted or diphasic in Lead III. In Lead aVR it is usually inverted, and in aVF it is usually upright. In Lead aVL the P wave may be in either direction.

In the chest leads V1 and V2 the P waves are usually diphasic, but in the other leads, the P waves are usually upright unless there is nodal rhythm.

1a. Idioventricular Rhythm.—This is an uncommon condition, in which there seems to be no supraventricular pacemaker and the ventricles beat at their own slower, inherent rate. No P waves are visible, and the QRS complexes may be

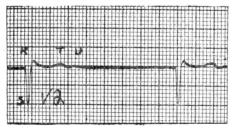

Fig. 47.—No P waves are visible. The ventricles are beating at their own inherent rate. Idioventricular rhythm. Note the slight abnormality of the ventricular component.

slightly abnormal and have some of the appearances of bundle-branch block due to abnormal conduction through ventricular muscle tissue. (*Fig.* 47.)

1*b*. Atrial Fibrillation.—This has been dealt with previously (*see* p. 20).

2. P Pulmonale.—This is a tall, peaked wave which may be up to 5 mm. high with little or no increase in duration. It is best seen in Leads II and III and may be due to: pulmonary hypertension from any cause but especially massive pulmonary embolism; pulmonary stenosis; tricuspid stenosis; tricuspid incompetence and cor pulmonale. (*Fig.* 48).

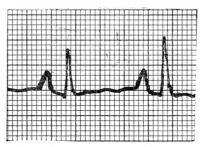

Fig. 48.—Tall, peaked P waves. P pulmonale.

3. P Mitrale.—This is a large, wide, and bifid P wave. The amplitude may be but slightly increased, but the duration may be up to 0·12 sec.

The first peak represents right atrial activity, the second left atrial activity, so that the bifid P mitrale implies delay in activation of the left atrium. It is best seen in Leads I and II and chest lead V5.

P mitrale is most often seen in mitral stenosis. (*Fig.* 49.)

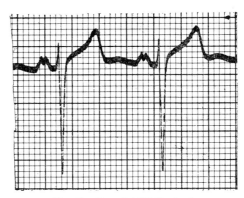

Fig. 49.—Broad, bifid P mitrale.

4. Inverted P Waves.—If present in most leads are suggestive of nodal rhythm (*see* p. 26).

If present in Lead I only, an inverted P wave is said to be suspicious of dextrocardia, but it can also occur if the leads are incorrectly placed on the wrong limbs.

An inverted P wave in chest lead V1 and sometimes in V2, may be physiological and inverted P waves in the limb leads II and III are very suggestive of coronary sinus rhythm.

5. Multiple P Waves.—

    a. Atrial flutter (*see* p. 21).

    b. Atrial fibrillation (*see* p. 20).

    c. Atrial tachycardia with atrioventricular block (*see* p. 17).

    d. Heart-block (*see* p. 24).

Having looked at the P wave in every lead and diagnosed any abnormalities which may be present, we pass on to Stage V.

STAGE V.—THE P–R INTERVAL

Examine the P–R *interval in every complex. If normal, pass on to Stage VI; if abnormal, consider the possible causes.*

The P–R interval varies normally from 0·10 sec. to 0·2 sec. It should be constant in every complex. The abnormalities to be considered are:—

1. Prolonged P–R Interval.—

This occurs in:—

    a. First-degree heart-block, which has already been dealt with on p. 24.

    b. Hyperkalaemia, which will be considered on p. 51.

    c. Other causes of prolonged P–R interval include:—

Diphtheria.

Digitalis therapy.

Acute rheumatic fever.

Arteriosclerosis.

Coronary occlusion, especially of the right coronary artery.

2. Short P–R Interval.—

    a. May be present in the *Wolff-Parkinson-White syndrome.* This is simply the presence of a short P–R interval, i.e., less than 0·08 sec., in association with bundle-branch block. It is usually congenital and is purely an electrocardiographic

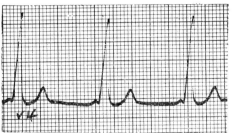

Fig. 50.—P–R interval 0·04 sec., associated with left bundle-branch block. Wolff-Parkinson-White syndrome.

diagnosis with little clinical significance, although it may precede paroxysmal tachycardia in some cases. (*Fig.* 50.)

It may be due to the premature excitation of one of the ventricles, as a result of an abnormal connexion between the atrioventricular node (or right atrium) and the right ventricle. Another theory is that it is due to accelerated conduction of a part of the excitatory process at the atrioventricular node.

The condition may be unstable and normal complexes may alternate with normal ones.

    b. Nodal Rhythm (*see* p. 26).

3. Variable P–R Interval.—*See* Wenckebach phenomenon, p. 25.

4. Complete P–R Dissociation of Third-degree Heart-block.—*See* p. 26.

Having considered the abnormalities of the P–R interval, we now pass on to the next stage.

STAGE VI.—THE Q WAVE

Examine the Q *wave in every lead.*

Q waves may normally be absent in some leads and can be deep in Lead V1.

The duration of the Q wave is not usually more than 0·04 sec. and it is usually 2 mm. or less in depth but will depend on the amplitude of the R–S complex. It should be not more than one-third of the amplitude of the R–S complex.

If pathological Q waves are present, i.e., deeper than 2 mm. or more than one-third the amplitude of the R–S complex, then we must consider the possibility of myocardial infarction.

I think it best to deal with the whole subject of myocardial infarction at this stage.

If only the inner part of the myocardium is affected, there will probably be no electrocardiographic changes. However, if the infarction involves the full thickness of the ventricle, characteristic changes will occur.

If the infarction spares the epicardium, i.e., if it is a 'sub-endocardial infarct', the only change may be the presence of deep, symmetrically inverted T waves.

Infarction of the anterolateral apical region of the left ventricle is usually due to occlusion of the left coronary artery or the left anterior descending branch.

Infarction of the posterobasal area of the left ventricle is usually due to occlusion of the right coronary artery or its posterior descending branch.

Infarction of the posterolateral area of the left ventricle is usually due to occlusion of the circumflex branch of the left coronary artery.

Since there is very little basic difference in the electrocardiographic pattern of myocardial infarction, wherever the site, I will deal with the changes of infarction *per se*.

I suggest that you look first in the *anterior limb leads*, i.e., Leads I and aVL. Changes here will often also be seen in the chest leads V1–V6 and will indicate *anterior infarction*.

Then look in the *posterior limb leads*, i.e., Leads III and aVF, for evidence of *posterior infarction*.

If it is a posterior lateral infarction, there may also be changes in Leads V5 and V6. However, remember that the posterior limb leads can be notoriously misleading, in that T wave inversion can be present in normal individuals in Leads III, aVF, and sometimes V1 and V2, so that inverted T waves alone cannot always be considered as diagnostic of infarction.

The essential diagnostic criteria, electrocardiographically speaking, for myocardial infarction are as follows:—

1. Recent Infarction.—

a. PATHOLOGICAL OR ABNORMAL Q WAVES, by which I mean a Q wave which is more than 2 mm. in depth or more than one-third of the R–S complex. However, note that in Lead III the Q wave can be deeper, depending on the height of the

41

R wave. The pathological Q wave is due to the transmission of negative intra-cavity potentials from the dead area of the myocardium.

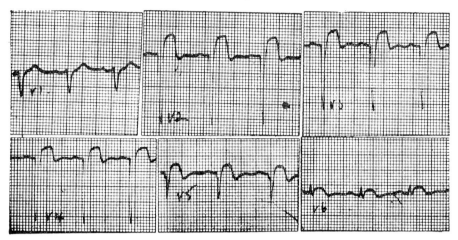

Fig. 51.—Recent extensive anterior infarction, stretching across the chest from leads V2 to V5.

b. S–T SEGMENT ELEVATION above the iso-electric axis. This elevated S–T segment in myocardial infarction is usually convex, which may help to differentiate it from the elevated S–T segment of pericarditis (*see* p. 55) which is often concave.

The S–T segment elevation reflects a current of injury arising from ischaemic damage to the epicardium around the infarcted area.

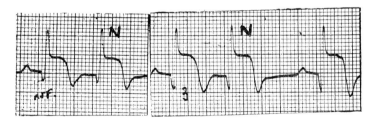

Fig. 52.—Recent posterior infarction with pathological Q waves and elevated S–T segments in the posterior limb leads. Note also the two complexes marked 'N' in which no P waves can be discerned. These are nodal ectopic beats and are followed by a compensatory pause.

These changes, viz., the pathological Q wave and the elevated S–T segment, are essential for the diagnosis of a recent myocardial infarction. They may appear a few hours after the infarct, but on occasions they may not show in the electrocardiogram for one or more days. (*Figs.* 51–53.)

If the electrocardiogram is taken shortly after the infarction has occurred the pathological Q wave may not yet be present and there will only be S–T segment elevation. However, the Q wave will usually appear within a few hours.

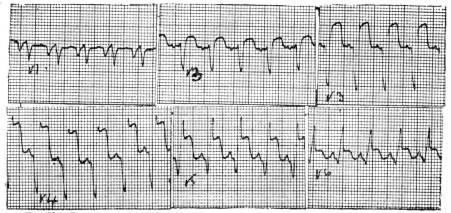

Fig. 53.—Recent anterior infarction. Elevated S–T segments extend right across the chest leads but pathological Q waves are not yet present in all leads. In Leads V1 to V3 small R waves still persist.

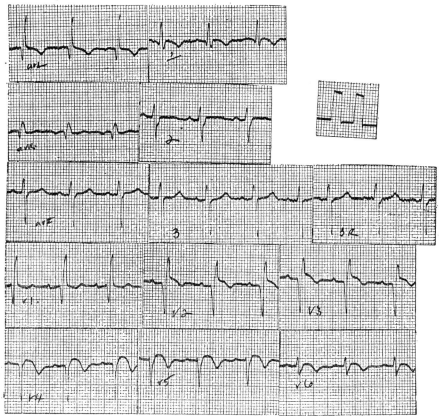

Fig. 54.—Regressive changes of anterior infarction. Pathological Q waves persist in anterior limb leads and in chest leads V1 to V4. The S–T segment has not yet had time to fall to the iso-electric line but it is on the way. There has been time for the T waves to become inverted.

43

In actual fact the S wave is frequently obscured in the presence of recent infarction and what is often loosely termed an S–T segment will be in reality a Q–T segment.

The infarction may be localized and evidenced only in Leads III and aVF if it is situated posteriorly. If more extensive and situated posterolaterally, abnormalities will also be seen in the lateral chest leads V6 and V5. Anterior infarcts may be limited to the septal area V2–V3 or may extend right across the chest from Lead V2 to V6 with changes occurring in limb leads I and aVL. In Lead III there may be S–T segment depression and the T wave may disappear.

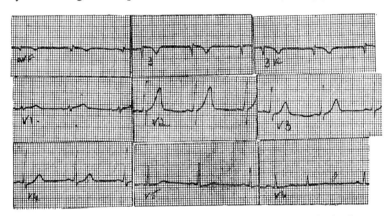

Fig. 55.—Regressive changes of posterior infarction. Q waves persist in the posterior limb leads. The S–T segment has become iso-electric and the T wave is inverted. The T waves are tall and peaked in chest leads V2 and V3.

2. Regressive Changes of Recent Myocardial Infarction.—After a variable time which may take from a few days to several weeks, the elevated S–T segment gradually drops back down towards the iso-electric line and will eventually become iso-electric. The T wave soon starts to become inverted and is often deepest by the time the S–T segment has reached the iso-electric axis. (*Figs. 54, 55.*)

The T wave inversion is due to reversal of the normal direction in which electrical recovery occurs. *If the* S–T *segment elevation persists after, say, three months, the possibility of ventricular aneurysm must be considered, as well as the likelihood of myocardial fibrosis.*

3. Old Infarction.—After some weeks, the inverted T wave usually becomes less marked but, nevertheless, may still be present. The pathological Q wave may be the only remaining evidence of old infarction and may persist indefinitely. (*Figs. 56, 57.*)

Remember that if these changes are seen in Leads I and aVL, the infarction is an anterior one and should be confirmed by looking at the chest leads which will often help to localize the site more accurately, so that an anteroseptal infarct shows changes maximal in the septal leads V2–V4 and an anterolateral infarct shows changes maximal in Leads V5 and V6 as well as in Leads I and aVL and sometimes Lead II. It is important to note that sometimes a typical anterior myocardial infarction may show up in the chest leads whilst there may be no evidence of it in the limb leads.

44

If the above changes are seen in Leads III and aVF, then the infarction is situated posteriorly, in which case changes may also sometimes occur to a lesser extent in Lead II.

I would emphasize that the diagnosis of myocardial infarction per se *is not sufficient and demands evaluation of its site, extent, and its stage of evolution in time.*

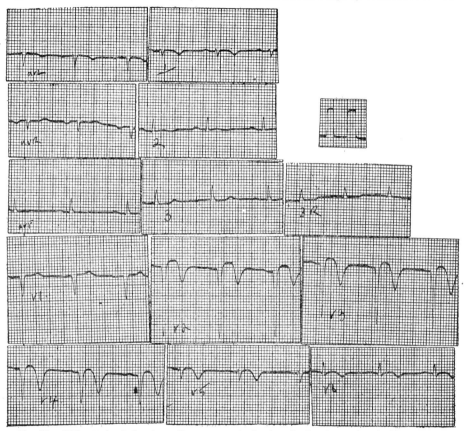

Fig. 56.—Old anterior infarction. Q waves persist in chest leads V1 to V4. The T waves are still deeply inverted in anterior limb leads and chest leads.

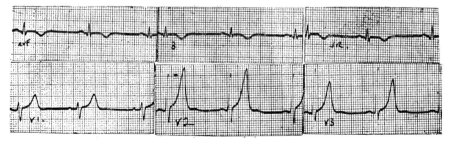

Fig. 57.—Old posterior infarction. Symmetrical T-wave inversion in posterior limb leads. Tall, peaked T waves in V2 and V3. Note that there are now no pathological Q waves.

STAGE VII.—THE QRS COMPLEX

Look at the QRS complex in every lead. If normal, pass on to Stage VIII; if abnormal, consider the possible causes:—
    1. Widening of the QRS complex.
        a. Bundle-branch block.
        b. High serum potassium.
        c. Ventricular ectopic beats.
        d. Quinidine.
        e. Ventricular hypertrophy.
    2. Low-voltage QRS complex.
        a. Hypothyroidism.
        b. Pericardial effusion.
        c. Chronic constrictive pericarditis.
        d. A thick chest wall.
        e. Myocardial infarction.
    3. Changes in shape of the QRS complex.
        a. In bundle-branch block producing slurring of R or S waves with widening of the complex and in right bundle-branch block, the presence of 'M' complexes.
        b. In acute cor pulmonale, the transient appearance of an S wave in Lead I, a Q wave in Lead III, S–T segment elevation in Lead aVR, and depression in Lead V6 and in some of the limb leads.
        c. Abnormal configuration in myocardial infarction.
        d. Ventricular tachycardia.
        e. Ventricular fibrillation.
        f. Ventricular flutter.
        g. Variation in axis deviation.
The normal duration of the QRS complex may be up to 0·11 sec. in adults and 0·045 sec. in infants, whilst in older children the duration may be up to 0·09 sec.
The QRS duration should be measured in the limb lead in which it is maximal.

1. Widening of the QRS Complex.—

a. BUNDLE-BRANCH BLOCK.—This is the most common abnormality of the QRS complex. As the name implies, it is the result of delay in conduction of the normal electrical impulse within one or other branches of the bundle of His. This delays contraction of the corresponding ventricle and excitation has to take place by slow muscle-to-muscle conduction from the other ventricle. It is mainly an electrocardiographic diagnosis but may be suspected clinically.

There are various types of bundle-branch block which are most simply classified as follows:—
    i. *Complete bundle-branch block.*
        α. Left.
        β. Right.

46

ii. *Incomplete bundle-branch block.*
  α. Left.
  β. Right.
iii. *Partial bundle-branch block.*
  α. Left.
  β. Right.
iv. *Wolff-Parkinson-White syndrome*, which is dealt with on p. 40.

i. COMPLETE BUNDLE-BRANCH BLOCK.—This implies a blockage of electrical conduction from the atrioventricular node through one of the branches of the bundle of His.

On the electrocardiogram, the duration of the QRS complex is prolonged above 0·12 sec. in the standard leads. There is frequently associated slurring and/or notching of R and/or S waves.

The T waves and P–R intervals are normal, suggesting that the conduction down as far as the atrioventricular node has followed the normal pathway. This helps in differentiating complete bundle-branch block from ventricular ectopic beats.

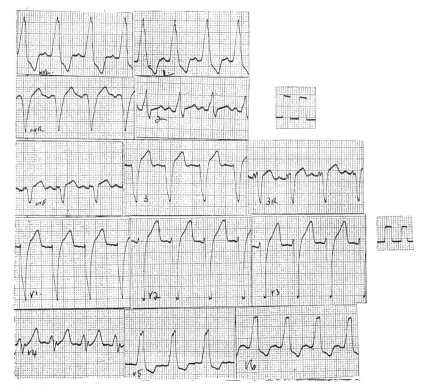

Fig. 58.—Complete left bundle-branch block. The QRS complexes have a prolonged duration—0·18–0·2 sec. Also, the R and S waves are notched and slurred, i.e., bundle-branch block is present. These changes are present in every complex in every lead so that the bundle-branch block is complete. In chest leads V1 and V6 the S wave in Lead V1 and the R wave in Lead V6 are the components most affected, i.e., there is left bundle-branch block.

α. *In left bundle-branch block*, the main deflexion (i.e., the deflexion of longest duration of the QRS complex) is upright in Leads I and aVL and is slurred. There is also, as mentioned previously, widening of the complex.

The longest duration of the QRS complex in Lead III is downwards or negative.

In the chest leads, the R wave in Leads V5 or V6 is large and wide and may be interrupted by a relatively early notch.

In Leads V1 and V2 there are small R waves and deep wide S waves and these changes are also seen in Leads III and aVF.

Left bundle-branch block is almost always indicative of organic heart disease and is especially seen in: hypertensive heart disease; ischaemic heart disease; aortic valve disease; myocarditis and cardiac fibrosis. (*Fig.* 58.)

β. *In right bundle-branch block* the part of the QRS complex of longest duration, i.e., the widest part, is deflected downwards in Lead I and upwards in Lead III, and is usually considerably deformed and slurred. Also, in Leads I and II, the T waves are opposite in direction to these main deflexions.

In the chest leads, the R waves in V1 and V2 and the S waves in V5 and V6 are most affected, and Leads V1 and V2 usually show a second R wave, resulting in a complex known as an R–S–R pattern or R_1R_2 pattern, or 'M wave' which is illustrated in *Fig.* 59 and is frequently associated with an inverted T wave.

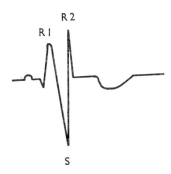

Fig. 59.—The 'M' complex of right bundle-branch block.

Usually, the changes in Leads V5 and V6 are transmitted to Leads I and aVL and the 'M' complex of Leads V1 to V2 is usually seen in Leads III and aVF.

Right bundle-branch block may occur in normal individuals and have no clinical significance. It may also be present in massive pulmonary embolus; atrial septal defect; mitral stenosis; ischaemic heart disease; and Ebstein's disease. (*Figs.* 60, 61.)

ii. INCOMPLETE BUNDLE-BRANCH BLOCK.—The duration of the QRS complex is longer than the normal 0.10 sec., but not as long as the 0·20 sec. of complete bundle-branch block. There is usually some slurring and notching of R and S waves.

When the QRS complexes are of low amplitude, the term 'arborization block' is used, implying defect of the electrical conduction in the small arbors of the Purkinje system.

iii. PARTIAL BUNDLE-BRANCH BLOCK.—This is uncommon and is said to be present when one normal QRS complex alternates with a complex showing

48

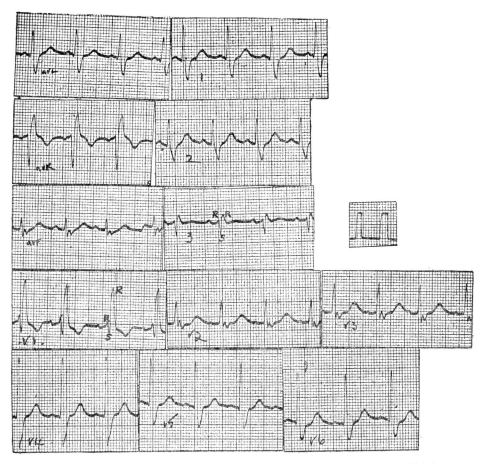

Fig. 60.—Complete right bundle-branch block. Note the typical R–S–R pattern (which is not usually present in all leads).

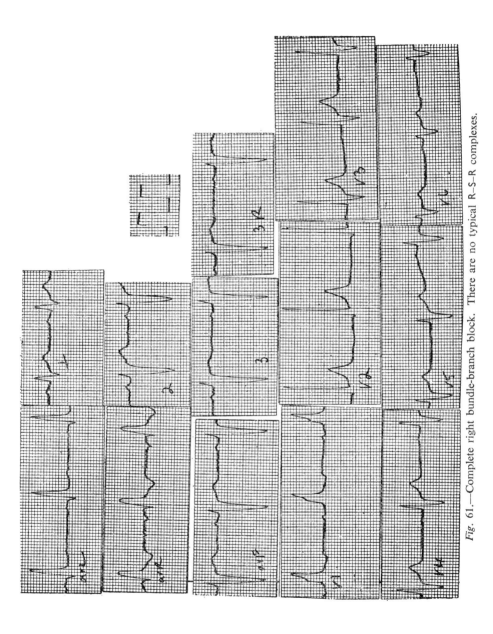

Fig. 61.—Complete right bundle-branch block. There are no typical R–S–R complexes.

50

bundle-branch block. This would be a 2 : 1 partial bundle-branch block, but 3 : 1 block, 4 : 1 block, and so on can occur. (*Fig.* 62.)

This situation may be difficult to differentiate from ventricular ectopic beats, but in the latter, there may be no P wave, or if there is, the P–R interval is shortened.

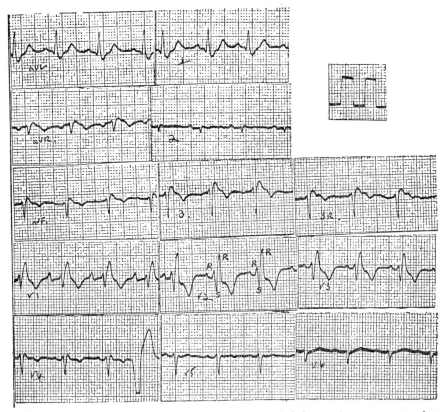

Fig. 62.—Partial right bundle-branch block. Typical R–S–R complexes are present but the changes are not seen in all leads; Leads II, V5, and V6 have no increase in QRS duration. Note electrical interference in Lead V6.

b. HIGH SERUM POTASSIUM.—The widening of the QRS complex in this condition is associated with a tall peaked T wave and sometimes with a diphasic QRS–T complex. Less often, the P–R interval may be prolonged. Often, not all of these changes are present together. (*Fig.* 63.)

Goldberger in 1962, in his book on *Water, Electrolyte and Acid-base Syndromes*, correlated the electrocardiographic picture with the serum potassium level. As a rough guide, when the serum potassium is between 6 and 7 mEq./l. the T waves are tall and peaked and have a narrow base. At 8 mEq./l. T waves may disappear or wander in and out of the QRS complex. At 10 mEq./l. wide aberrant QRS complexes with diphasic deflexions occur caused by fusion of the QRS complex, the RS–T segment, and the T wave. At 12 mEq./l. there usually results ventricular fibrillation and cardiac standstill.

51

c. VENTRICULAR ECTOPIC BEATS.—These have been discussed on p. 29.

d. QUINIDINE.—This tends to depress the electrical activity in the heart. The duration of the QRS complex and of the P wave is increased. The T wave is depressed, slurred, and widened, and the duration of the Q-T interval is increased.

2. Low-voltage QRS Complex.—This is often associated with flattened or inverted T waves in both myxoedema and chronic constrictive pericarditis. In myxoedema there will usually be an associated sinus bradycardia. The whole tracing is of low amplitude (*Fig.* 64), the QRS complex rarely reaching 6 mm.

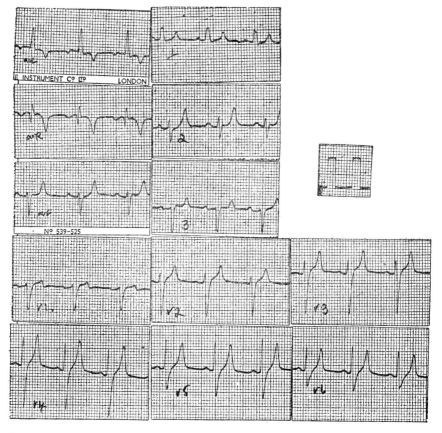

Fig. 63.—High serum potassium. Tall spiky T waves in almost every lead with widening and slurring of the QRS complexes in some leads.

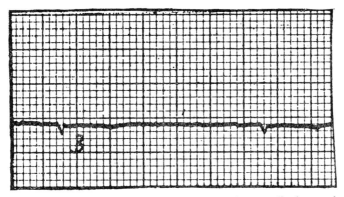

Fig. 64.—Myxoedema. Sinus bradycardia with very low amplitude complexes.

STAGE VIII.—THE Q–T INTERVAL

Examine the Q–T *interval in every complex. If it is normal, pass on to Stage IX.*

The Q–T interval includes the interval between the beginning of the QRS complex and the end of the T waves and will vary directly with age and sex, and inversely with the cardiac rate so that it is shorter in the presence of tachycardia and vice versa. The normal Q–T interval is up to 0·4 sec.

For this reason a true evaluation of the Q–T interval requires a correction for cardiac rate. This is done simply by 'Bazett's formula':—

$$\text{Q–T (corrected)} = \frac{\text{Q–T interval}}{\sqrt{\text{R–R}}} \quad \text{(i.e., length of cardiac cycle)}$$

e.g., in *Fig.* 65 the Q–T interval is 0·24 sec. Length of cardiac cycle is 0·32 sec.

$$\therefore \ \text{Q–T (corrected)} = \frac{0·25}{\sqrt{0·32}} = \frac{0·25}{0·57} = 0·43 \text{ sec.}$$

The Q–T interval is prolonged in: hypocalcaemia; active rheumatic carditis; cardiac enlargment; myocardial ischaemia; and diphtheritic heart disease.

It is shortened in digitalis therapy and hypercalcaemia.

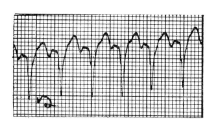

Fig. 65.—Measured Q–T interval is 0·24 sec. Q–T interval corrected for rate is 0·43 sec.

STAGE IX.—THE S–T SEGMENT

Examine the S–T *segment in every complex. If it is normal, pass on to Stage X, and if abnormal, consider the following causes:—*

1. The S–T segment may be elevated in:—
   a. Recent myocardial infarction.
   b. Pericarditis.
   c. Slight S–T segment elevation up to 1 mm. may be normal in chest leads V1 and V2.
   d. Cardiac trauma.
   e. Hyperkalaemia.

2. The S–T segment may be depressed in:—
   a. Ischaemia.
   b. Digitalis therapy.
   c. Tachycardia.
   d. Hypokalaemia.
   e. Ventricular hypertrophy.
   f. Bundle-branch block.
   g. Ventricular ectopic beats.

Recent Myocardial Infarction.—The S–T segment elevation of recent myocardial infarction has already been discussed. Remember that it must be associated with the presence of a pathological Q wave, although this may be a little slower in developing. (*See* p. 42.)

Pericarditis.—In the early stages of all types of pericarditis except in the presence of an effusion, the RS–T segment will be elevated. However, there will be no pathological Q waves so that usually the differentiation from recent myocardial infarction is not difficult. Also, as mentioned previously, the elevated RS–T

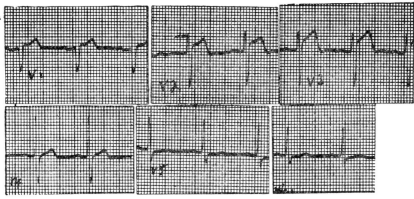

Fig. 66.—Pericarditis. The S–T segments in chest leads V2 and V3 (and to a lesser extent in Lead V1) denote an area of localized pericarditis.

segment of pericarditis is often concave, whereas in recent myocardial infarction it is usually convex.

After a few days the elevated RS–T segment begins to fall towards the iso-electric level and at a later stage still the T waves become inverted.

If the pericarditis is generalized, these changes will appear in all leads. However, pericarditis is often localized over a small area of the heart and the changes will then be seen only in the relevant leads of the electrocardiogram. Localized pericarditis is probably most commonly seen in the very early stages of myocardial infarction, although it may arise some days later in the so-called post-myocardial infarction or 'Dressler's syndrome'. If there is an effusion, the QRS complexes are of low voltage. (*Figs.* 66, 67.)

CHRONIC CONSTRICTIVE PERICARDITIS.—In this condition the QRS complexes may be of low voltage, but the most important electrocardiographic change is generalized inversion or flattening of the T waves. Sometimes the T waves are prominent and widened.

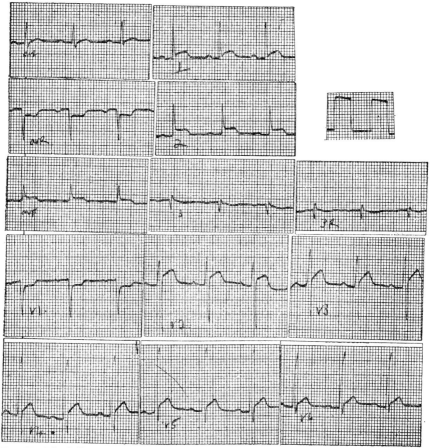

Fig. 67.—The S–T segments are elevated in Leads I, II, III, aVF, IIIR, and in all the chest leads.

Ischaemia and Digitalis Effect.—In myocardial ischaemia the S–T segment may be depressed, but there is not infrequently a normal electrocardiogram in a patient with a history of angina pectoris. The electrocardiographic changes can be brought out in this situation by taking a tracing after exercise. However, this can be a dangerous procedure! There may also be present inversion of the U wave in both of these conditions. (*Figs.* 68, 69.)

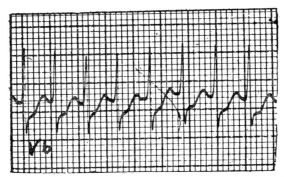

Fig. 68.—Ischaemia—in this case due to the marked tachycardia.

Digitalis therapy can also give rise to depression of the S–T segment and this depression is difficult to differentiate from that of ischaemia. However, it is often said that the depression or sag of the S–T segment in myocardial ischaemia is

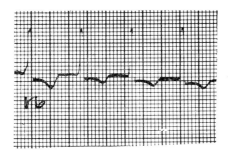

Fig. 69.—Severe ischaemia producing S–T segment depression and T-wave inversion.

gradual and has a gradually curved return towards the iso-electric axis (*Fig.* 70). In digitalis therapy the S–T segment looks as if it has been pulled downwards and it has a much sharper return towards the iso-electric line (*Fig.* 71). Since either of these appearances may be seen in either condition, I do not think that this point is of much help in differentiation. However, it may help to note that ischaemic changes *may* be restricted whereas digitalis usually produces changes in every lead. (*Fig.* 72.)

We can see from previous sections that digitalis has numerous effects on the myocardium and vagus nerve which may be manifested electrocardiographically. These changes include: bradycardia; S–T segment depression; heart-block; bigeminus or occasional ventricular ectopic beats; nodal rhythm; shortening of the corrected Q–T interval. These changes are usually seen in all leads, but are especially prominent in Leads II and V5.

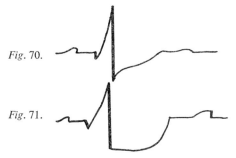

Fig. 70.

Fig. 71.

Fig. 70.—The electrocardiogram in myocardial ischaemia showing gradually curved return of S–T segment to iso-electric axis.

Fig. 71.—The electrocardiogram in digitalis therapy showing a sharper return of S–T segment to iso-electric axis.

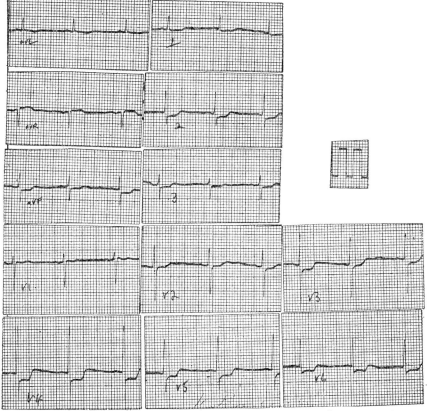

Fig. 72.—Digitalis effect with S–T segment depression in almost every complex. Rate: 75 beats per min.

STAGE X.—THE T WAVE

Examine the T *wave in every complex.*

It varies considerably in size, but is usually more than 2 mm. high and is usually upright in all leads, although it can be inverted in limb leads III and aVR, chest lead V1, and less often V2.

If the T wave is normal, we have almost completed the systematic examination of our electrocardiographic tracing and it will remain only to consider a few miscellaneous conditions.

If the T wave is abnormal, we must consider the possible reasons:—

1. *Tall, peaked* T *waves.*—

a. High serum potassium—this has already been dealt with on p. 51.

b. In posterior infarction the T waves may be tall and peaked in some of the chest leads, as dealt with on p. 44.

2. *Flattened* T *waves.*—

a. Hypothyroidism—this has already been dealt with on p. 52.

b. Pericarditis—this has already been dealt with on p. 55.

c. Ischaemia.

3. *Inverted* T *waves.*—

a. Severe myocardial ischaemia.

b. Pericarditis.

c. Low serum potassium.

d. Ventricular hypertrophy.

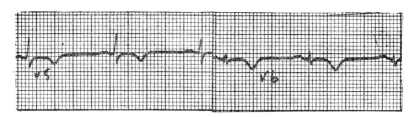

Fig. 73.—Symmetrical T-wave inversion suspicious of old infarction.

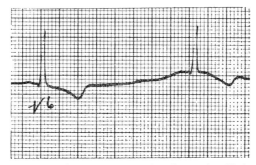

Fig. 74.—Asymmetrical T-wave inversion diagnostic of ischaemia.

5*

Severe myocardial ischaemia may produce T-wave inversion which can be quite marked. This may, of course, coexist with depression of the S–T segment (*see Fig.* 69, p. 57).

Many people diagnose infarction on the basis of severe T-wave inversion, others interpret this as merely ischaemia. It is said that if the T-wave inversion is symmetrical, infarction is more likely (*Fig.* 73); asymmetrical T-wave inversion is said to be more typical of ischaemia. (*Fig.* 74.)

b. Constrictive pericarditis (*see* p. 56).

c. Low serum potassium.

d. Ventricular hypertrophy.

The inverted T wave usually occurs in every lead when due to hypokalaemia and is associated with prominent U waves and a prolonged P–R interval. (*Fig.* 75.) Initially the T wave may merely be flattened.

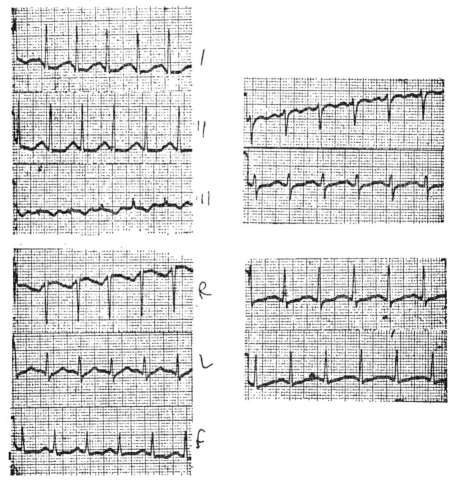

Fig. 75.—Sinus tachycardia with flattening of T waves in all leads and slight S–T segment depression. There is a prominent late wave resulting from U–P fusion. Hypokalaemia.

We have now considered almost all of the possible diagnoses which can be made by use of the electrocardiogram alone. However, one condition does not fit happily into any one of the categories listed, and so must be dealt with separately. This is the picture of *pulmonary embolism.*

Not all pulmonary emboli produce electrocardiographic changes; however, in a classic case with a massive pulmonary embolus, some or all of the following changes may appear:—

1. A deep S wave in Lead I associated with a pathological Q wave and an inverted T wave in Lead III.

2. Tall, peaked P waves (or P pulmonale) which may be present in any lead, but occur especially in chest leads V1 and V2.

3. Right axis deviation.

4. Incomplete right bundle-branch block.

5. Inverted T waves in chest leads V1 and V2.

6. S–T segment sag in chest leads V5 and V6. (*Figs.* 76, 77.)

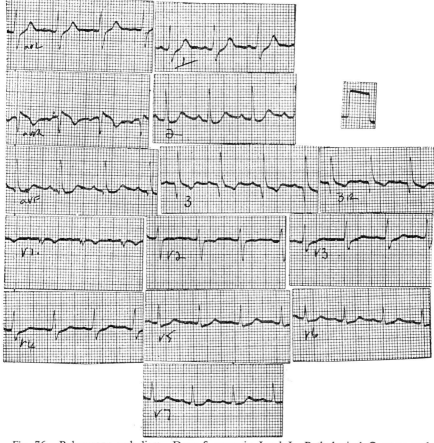

Fig. 76.—Pulmonary embolism. Deep S wave in Lead I. Pathological Q wave and inverted T wave in Lead III. Inverted T waves in Leads V1 and V2. Slight S–T sag in Leads V5 and V6.

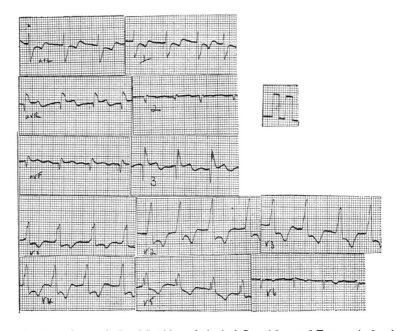

Fig. 77.—Deep S wave in Lead I with pathological Q and inverted T waves in Lead III. Right axis deviation. Incomplete bundle-branch block (right). Inverted T waves over right ventricular leads. S–T segment sag over left ventricle. Pulmonary embolus.

CHAPTER III

ARTEFACTS

HAVING discussed much of the information which may be gained by careful interpretation of an electrocardiogram, I would mention that there are some conditions which can produce concern and lead to misinterpretation.

1. Electrical Interference.—Some of the newer transistorized machines run exclusively by battery, so that electrical interference is no problem, but most machines at present in use run from the electricity supply and are prone to pick up electrical interference in the form of a regular wave pattern of 50 or 60 cycles per sec. This can often be stopped by switching off any electrical appliances running on the same circuit. Sometimes, connecting the machine by an earthing wire to a metal water tap can help. (*Fig.* 78.)

2. Somatic Tremor.—This is due to skeletal muscle contraction and occurs especially when the patient is nervous or cold. It results in rapid irregular low voltage vibration which distorts all the electrocardiographic complexes. (*Fig.* 79.)

3. Movement of the Patient.—This produces sudden upward or downward deflexion. (*Fig.* 80.)

4. Shifting of the Base-line.—This can be due to loose contacts in any place in the circuit or cutaneous current and can also be due to the swinging of loose wires conducting electricity if they are close to the electrocardiographic leads. It can produce a false impression of S–T segment sag or elevation. (*Fig.* 81.)

Sufficient abrasion with electrode jelly and careful connexion of lead to contact prevent most cases of shifting base-line.

5. Incorrect Connexions.—If the incorrect leads are connected to uncorresponding electrodes, a completely unreliable tracing may result, so that it is important to join up the left-arm lead to the left arm, the left-leg lead to the left leg, and so on.

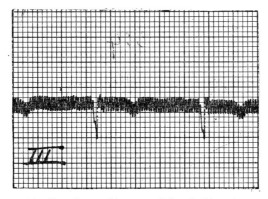

Fig. 78.—Regular, rapid waves of electrical interference.

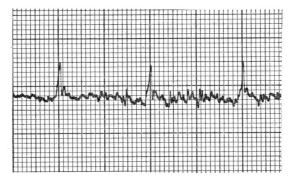

Fig. 79.—Rapid, uneven, and irregular waves due to somatic muscle tremor.

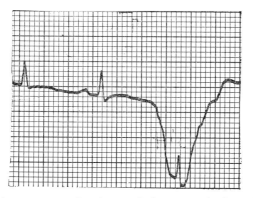

Fig. 80.—Sudden movement of patient producing an erratic change in the tracing.

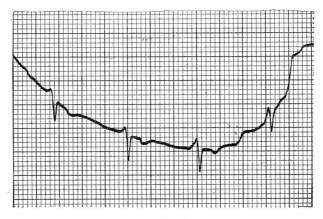

Fig. 81.—Shifting base-line.

APPENDIX

THE following electrocardiograms, with their commentaries, will help to illustrate the points in the preceding pages.

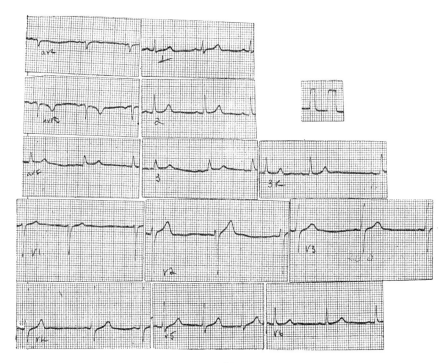

Fig. 82.

Stage I—Rate approximately 75 beats per min.
Stage II—Rhythm is regular.
Stage III—Axis deviation, etc.—no relevant comments.
Stage IV—P waves are normal.
Stage V—P–R interval is normal.
Stage VI—There are no pathological Q waves.
Stage VII—The QRS complexes are normal.
Stage VIII—There is no abnormality of the S–T segments.
Stage IX—The S–T segments are normal.
Stage X—The T waves are normal.
Summary—A normal electrocardiogram.

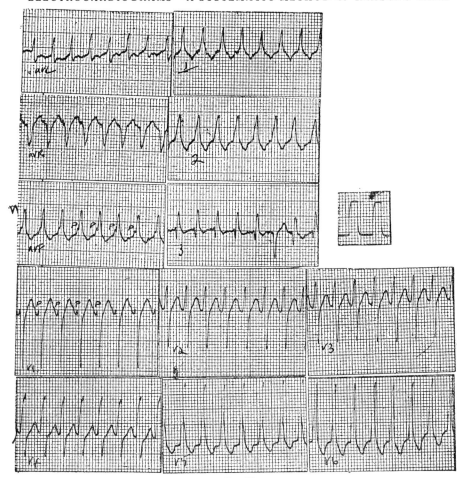

Fig. 83.

Stage I—The rate is approximately 230 beats per min. The complexes look fairly normal so that this is a supraventricular tachycardia. It is difficult to differentiate here between atrial and nodal tachycardia, but in some leads, e.g., aVF and V1, P waves can be seen merging with the rest of the complex because of the gross tachycardia. Probably atrial tachycardia.

Stage II—The rhythm is regular apart from an occasional ectopic beat (Lead III) which is quite bizarre compared with other complexes in the same lead, i.e., a ventricular ectopic beat.

Stage III—No relevant axis deviation.

Stage IV—The P waves are difficult to discern, being merged with the other complexes in most leads.

Stage V—The P–R interval is similarly difficult to define.

Stage VI—There are no pathological Q waves.

Stage VII—The QRS complexes are almost normal, taking into account the very rapid rate. However, the S waves in V1 are deep and the R waves in V6 are tall and, in fact, the sum of S in V1 and R in V6 is 36 mm., i.e., there is left ventricular hypertrophy.

Stage VIII—The Q–T interval is normal.

Stage IX—There is slight S–T segment sag in many leads, suggesting ischaemia associated with the marked tachycardia.

66

Stage X—T-wave inversion similarly is due to ischaemia and possibly to some extent to left ventricular hypertrophy.

Summary—Atrial tachycardia with an occasional ventricular ectopic beat and associated ischaemia. Left ventricular hypertrophy.

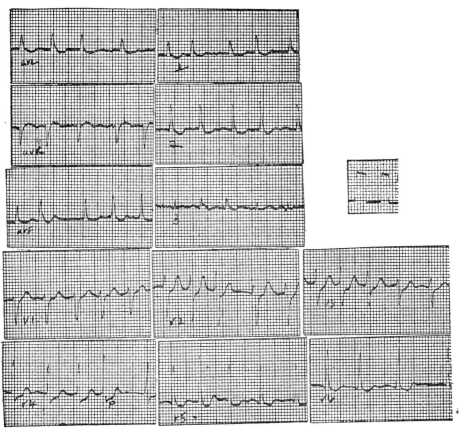

Fig. 84.

Stage I—The rate is approximately 150 beats per min.

Stage II—The rhythm is completely irregular. Why? A large number of ectopic beats can be seen which look fairly normal and are therefore likely to be supraventricular in origin. Some of these ectopics, e.g., in Lead V4, are seen to have the P wave merged in with the T wave. In other ectopic complexes no P wave can be made out, i.e., there are multiple nodal and ectopic beats.

Stage III—No relevant axis deviation.

Stage IV and *Stage V*—The P waves and P–R interval are normal, apart from the comments above.

Stage VI—There are no pathological Q waves.

Stage VII—The QRS complexes are normal.

Stage VIII—The Q–T intervals are normal.

Stage IX—There is S–T segment depression due to ischaemia associated with the tachycardia.

Stage X—The T waves are normal.

Summary—Tachycardia due to multiple nodal ectopic beats with resulting ischaemia.

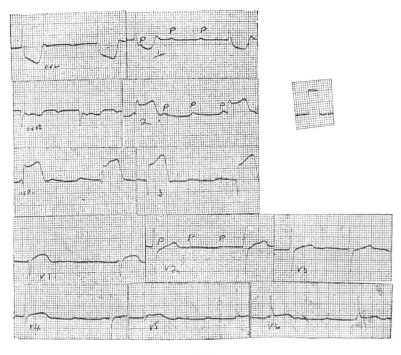

Fig. 85.

Stage I—The ventricular rate is approximately 40 beats per min. However, three P waves can be discerned for every QRS complex, i.e., there is 3 : 1 atrioventricular block. The P–R interval is different for each complex, i.e., there is *complete* 3 : 1 atrioventricular block.

Stage II—The rhythm is regular.

Stage III—There is left axis deviation, but no hypertrophy.

Stage IV and *Stage V*—The P waves and P–R interval have been discussed.

Stage VI—There are pathological Q waves in Lead III and in both posterior limb leads and in Lead II there are elevated S–T segments, i.e., there has been a recent extensive posterior infarction.

Stage VII—There are no other abnormalities of the QRS complexes.

Stage VIII—The Q–T interval is normal.

Stage IX—The S–T segment is considerably depressed in Leads I and aVL. This is purely reciprocal to the elevation already discussed in Leads III and aVF.

Stage X—The T wave is normal apart from its association with the S–T segments as discussed above.

Summary—Complete 3 : 1 atrioventricular block. Recent extensive posterior infarction.

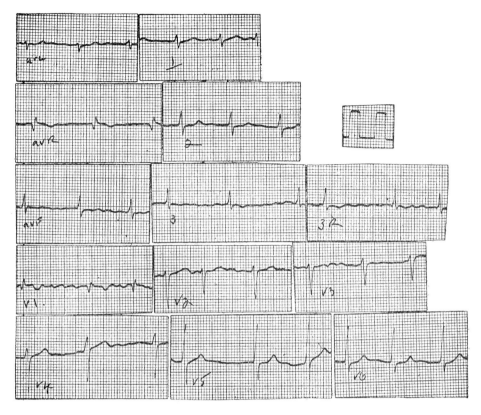

Fig. 86.

Stage I—The rate is approximately 70 beats per min.

Stage II—The rhythm is completely irregular. Also 'f' waves can be easily made out especially in Leads V1, V3, and in all the posterior limb leads. In the other leads the P waves bear a variable relationship to the QRS complexes. Atrial fibrillation.

Stage III—There is slight axis deviation. In association with this the S waves are rather prominent in left ventricular leads so that there is some degree of right ventricular dominance.

Stage IV and *Stage V*—The P waves and P–R interval have been discussed.

Stage VI—There are no pathological Q waves.

Stage VII—The QRS complexes are normal apart from the slightly prominent S waves over the left ventricular leads discussed above.

Stage VIII—The Q–T interval is normal.

Stage IX and *Stage X*—The S–T segments and T waves are normal.

Summary—Atrial fibrillation. Slight right ventricular dominance.

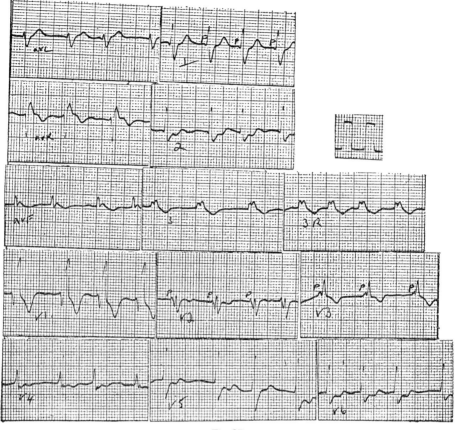

Fig. 87.

Stage I—The rate is approximately 110 beats per min.

Stage II—The rhythm is regular apart from occasional atrial and nodal ectopic beats.

Stage III—Axis deviation is difficult to define in the presence of obvious QRS complex abnormality.

Stage IV—The P waves are small and often difficult to make out.

Stage V—The P–R interval is very short—best seen in Leads I and V3.

Stage VI—The Q wave is normal.

Stage VII—The QRS complexes are wide—over 0·12 sec., i.e., there is bundle-branch block. However, not all the complexes are abnormally wide, e.g., those in Leads aVF, V3, and V4 are of normal duration, i.e., the bundle-branch block is only partial. In Leads V1 and V6, the R wave of V1 and the S wave of V6 are most affected. Therefore, it is right bundle-branch block.

Stage VIII—The Q–T interval is normal.

Stage IX and *Stage X*—The S–T segment is a little depressed in some leads and the T wave inverted—as may occur with right bundle-branch block. There is also present some ischaemic change.

Summary—Occasional atrial and nodal ectopic beats. Short P–R interval plus partial right bundle-branch block—Wolff-Parkinson-White syndrome.

70

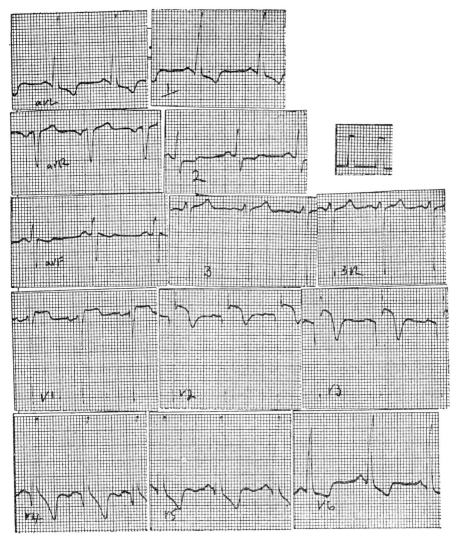

Fig. 88.

Stage I—Rate is 75 beats per min. approximately.

Stage II—The rhythm is regular.

Stage III—There is marked left axis deviation and left ventricular hypertrophy.

Stage IV and *Stage V*—The P waves and P–R interval are normal.

Stage VI—There are pathological Q waves across the chest leads from V2 to V4. These are associated with elevation of the S–T (or more correctly Q–S) segments, i.e., there has been a recent anterior infarction. However, the S–T segment is falling and the T waves are inverted, so regressive changes are occurring.

Stage VII—The QRS duration is at the upper limit of normal in some leads. There is partial left bundle-branch block.

Stage VIII—The Q–T interval is normal.

71

Stage IX—The S–T segment has been considered.

Stage X—The gross T-wave inversion is associated with marked left ventricular hypertrophy.

Summary—Left ventricular hypertrophy. Recent anteroseptal infarction. Partial left bundle-branch block.

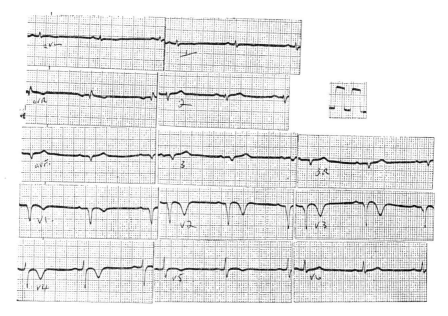

Fig. 89.

Stage I—Rate is just under 60 beats per min. The P waves and P–R interval are normal. Sinus bradycardia.

Stage II—The rhythm is regular.

Stage III—Slight left axis deviation but no hypertrophy.

Stage IV and *Stage V*—The P wave and P–R interval are normal.

Stage VI—Pathological Q waves are present in chest leads V1 to V3. However, the S–T segment is iso-electric but the T waves are deeply inverted. This T-wave inversion extends across to V5. Old anterolateral infarction.

Stage VII—The QRS complexes are normal but of large amplitude and associated with brady-cardia; suggest myxoedema.

Stage VIII—The Q–T intervals are normal.

Stage IX—The S–T segments are normal.

Stage X—The T waves have been considered.

Summary—An extensive, old anterolateral infarction. Possible myxoedema.

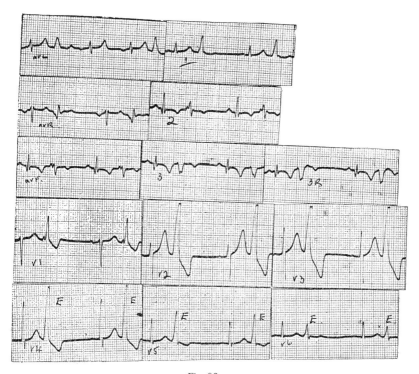

Fig. 90.

Stage I—Rate is difficult to assess because of the irregularity. On the average it is about 80 beats per min.

Stage II—The rhythm is irregular. There are numerous ectopic beats, all of which are bizarre in shape and are therefore ventricular in origin. It will be noted that each ventricular ectopic beat is coupled with a normal beat—bigeminus or coupling.

Stage III—No significant axis deviation.

Stage IV and *Stage V*—The P waves and P–R interval are normal.

Stage VI—There are pathological Q waves in the posterior limb leads. These are associated with inverted T waves—old posterior infarction—substantiated by the peaked T waves in Leads V2 and V3.

Stage VII—The QRS complexes are normal, apart from the ectopic beats, of course.

Stage VIII—The Q–T interval is normal.

Stage IX—The S–T segment is normal.

Stage X—The T wave has been discussed in the posterior limb leads. It is normal in others.

Summary—Bigeminus—probably due to digoxin. Old posterior infarction.

73

INDEX